500 MCQs FOR THE MRCP PART 1

Titles of related interest from WB Saunders:

For MRCP examinations

Davies et al.	Modern Medicine for the MRCP	1996	07020 21121
Baliga	250 Short Cases in Clinical Medicine	1996	07020 22055
King	Picture Tests and Short Cases for the MRCP	1996	07020 18155
Galvani	Haematology for the MRCP	1995	07020 1883X
Elliott et al.	Pass the MRCP Parts I and II	1996	07020 21989

For practical use

Banerjee	Accident & Emergency Medicine: A Survival Guide	1996	07020 22101
Raby	Accident & Emergency Radiology: A Survival Guide	1995	07020 19054

500 MCQs FOR THE MRCP PART 1

RAGAVENDRA R BALIGA
MBBS MD DNB MRCP
Department of Medicine
Cardiovascular Division
Boston Medical Center
Boston, MA, USA

formerly of the Hammersmith
Hospital, London

WB SAUNDERS COMPANY LTD
LONDON   PHILADELPHIA   TORONTO
SYDNEY   TOKYO

W.B. Saunders Company Ltd   24–28 Oval Road
London NW1 7DX

The Curtis Center
Independence Square West
Philadelphia, PA 19106-3399, USA

Harcourt Brace & Company
55 Horner Avenue
Toronto, Ontario M8Z 4X6, Canada

Harcourt Brace & Company, Australia
30–52 Smidmore Street
Marrickville, NSW 2204, Australia

Harcourt Brace & Company, Japan
Ichibancho Central Building,
22-1 Ichibancho
Chiyoda-ku, Tokyo 102, Japan

A catalogue record for this book is available from the British Library

ISBN 0–7020–2243–8

Typeset by LaserScript, Mitcham, Surrey
Printed and bound in Great Britain by
WBC Book Manufacturers, Bridgend, Mid Glamorgan

CONTENTS

FOREWORD

Taking and passing postgraduate medical examinations is one of the dreaded hurdles for aspiring physicians who wish to pursue a career in internal medicine. On such examinations, multiple choice questions are frequently used to determine whether candidates understand and are able to apply essential facts. Merely reading medical textbooks may not adequately prepare the candidate for these examinations. This book, with 500 questions and detailed answers, is not intended to be a comprehensive reference text, but rather, to provoke thought, expose hidden areas of weakness and act as an aid in the preparation for postgraduate examinations. Used in this way, Dr. Baliga's book will be an invaluable supplement to traditional bedside and textbook teaching.

Wilson S. Colucci, MD, FACC
Chief, Cardiovascular Division
Boston Medical Center
Professor of Medicine
Boston University School of Medicine
Boston, Massachusetts
USA

PREFACE

This book consists of 500 multiple-choice questions designed to provide a comprehensive and useful review for those preparing for the MRCP Part 1 examination. The basic question types are in format for this examination: each statement or stem has five items, and the answer to each item is independent of every other item. While testing yourself you must decide on one of three options, viz., 'True', 'False' or 'Don't know'. Each question is accompanied by an answer, sometimes quite detailed. By allowing two and a half minutes for each stem, the time constraints of the MRCP examination may be simulated.

I thank Dr Wilson Colucci, Professor of Medicine for writing the Foreword and for his support.

I wish to thank Rachael Stock, Senior Editor, W.B. Saunders for inviting me to write this book. I also thank Heather Burroughs, the production editor of this book.

I once again support my wife Jayashree for doing my share of the domestic chores while I wrote this book.

RRB

Dedicated to the memory of my father

RAMAKRISHNA BALIGA, BE, DIISc, MBA (Paris)

who founded the Electronic City in Bangalore, India

1 CARDIOVASCULAR MEDICINE

1. *A 30-year-old male with a heart murmur underwent cardiac catheterization and the pressures (mmHg) were as follows: right atrium, 5; right ventricle, 60/0; pulmonary artery, 60/30; mean pulmonary artery wedge, 20; and left ventricle, 120/0. This patient has*

   A. mitral regurgitation.
   B. loud first heart sound.
   C. mid-diastolic rumbling murmur at the apex.
   D. opening snap.
   E. aortic stenosis.

   A........... B.......... C.......... D.......... E..........

2. *A 33-year-old lawyer complains of chest pain and giddiness on climbing stairs. His 29-year-old brother recently died during a long-distance running competition. Electrocardiogram excluded myocardial infarction but cardiac catheterization showed left ventricular pressures of 170/20 mmHg.*

   A. The patient has dilated cardiomyopathy.
   B. Echocardiography shows systolic anterior motion of the anterior mitral valve leaflet.
   C. The patient has diastolic dysfunction.
   D. There is asymmetric septal hypertrophy on echocardiography.
   E. The patient may have a double apical impulse.

   A........... B.......... C.......... D.......... E..........

3. *A 28-year-old asymptomatic man's electrocardiogram showed incomplete right bundle branch block and cardiac catheterization revealed the following oxygen saturation values (%): superior vena cava, 67; inferior vena cava, 64; right atrium, 82; right ventricle, 81; pulmonary artery, 81; left atrium, 96; left ventricle 96; and femoral artery, 94. Pressures (mmHg) were: right atrium, 9; right ventricle, 30/0; pulmonary artery, 30/10; left atrium, 10; left ventricle, 110/0; and femoral artery, 110/60.*

   A. This patient has a ventricular septal defect.
   B. On auscultation the patient has a wide fixed split second sound.
   C. This patient has an ostium primum defect of the atrial septum.
   D. The patient has undergone Eisenmenger's syndrome.
   E. Reversal of shunt occurs in the second decade.

   A........... B.......... C.......... D.......... E..........

1.   A. F   B. T   C. T   D. T   E. F

This patient has mitral stenosis which is characterised by a loud first heart sound, opening snap and a mid-diastolic rumbling murmur at the apex.

2.   A. F   B. T   C. T   D. T   E. T

This patient has hypertrophic cardiomyopathy. In approximately half the patients with hypertrophic cardiomyopathy the disease is familial and the pattern autosomal dominant with variable expression. Genes that have been implicated include those for β-myosin heavy chain, α-tropomyosin and troponin T. These patients have shortness of breath, syncope, angina pectoris, palpitations and sudden death. ECG may show left ventricular hypertrophy, deep Q waves and conduction defects. Electrocardiogram shows asymmetrical septal hypertrophy, systolic anterior motion of the mitral valve and mitral regurgitation. The course is extremely variable. The frequency of sudden death is 2–3% per year for adults. Differential diagnoses of diastolic dysfunction include amyloidosis and hypertensive heart disease coupled with age-related subaortic septal hypertrophy.

3.   A. F   B. T   C. F   D. T   E. T

This patient has an ostium secundum atrial septal defect. There is a left-to-right shunt at the atrial level with normal left and right heart haemodynamics. On auscultation, the patient will have a wide fixed split second sound. Ostium secundum defects account for 70% of the cases; the defect is in the middle portion of the atrial septum and is usually 2–4 cm in diameter and ECG shows incomplete right bundle branch block with the QRS axis rightward. Sinus venosus defect is located just below the entrance of the superior vena cava into the right atrium and ECG shows leftward P-wave axis so that P waves are inverted in at least one inferior lead. The ostium primum type is a defect in the lower part of the septum and clefts may occur in the mitral and tricuspid valves and the QRS axis is leftward. Reversal of shunt or Eisenmenger's syndrome usually occurs in the second decade.

4. *A 7-year-old child with a murmur underwent cardiac catheterization and the data obtained were as follows. Oxygen saturation (%): superior vena cava, 65; inferior vena cava, 65; right atrium, 87; right ventricle, 89; pulmonary artery, 90; and femoral artery, 96. Pressures (mmHg): right atrium, 3; right ventricle, 59/0; pulmonary artery, 16/8; and femoral artery, 105/65. This patient has*

    A. Fallot's tetralogy.
    B. aortic stenosis.
    C. aortic regurgitation.
    D. atrial septal defect.
    E. pulmonary stenosis.

    A...........   B..........   C..........   D..........   E..........

5. *Infective bacterial endocarditis*

    A. is usually caused by Gram-negative bacilli.
    B. when acute requires empiric antimicrobial treatment before culture report becomes available.
    C. when subacute is most often caused by staphylococci.
    D. caused by *Streptococcus bovis* is associated with lower gastrointestinal neoplasms.
    E. involving the tricuspid valve is seen most frequently in parenteral drug abusers.

    A...........   B..........   C..........   D..........   E..........

6. *The following statements about the treatment of bacterial endocarditis are correct.*

    A. Penicillin therapy results in a cure rate of less than half in subacute bacterial endocarditis caused by streptococci.
    B. Penicillin plus an aminoglycoside are the treatment of choice for enterococcal endocarditis.
    C. *Staphylococcus aureus* endocarditis should be treated with cloxacillin.
    D. In *Staphylococcus epidermidis* endocarditis, cephalosporins should be used to treat methicillin-resistant strains.
    E. In well-established bacterial endocarditis, therapy should not be initiated when blood cultures remain negative.

    A...........   B..........   C..........   D..........   E..........

7. *Indications for surgery in bacterial endocarditis include*

    A. fungal endocarditis refractory to medical therapy.
    B. prosthetic valve with non-streptococcal endocarditis.
    C. refractory heart failure.
    D. development of a new aneurysm of the sinus of Valsalva.
    E. drainage of a myocardial abscess.

    A...........   B..........   C..........   D..........   E..........

4.   A. F   B. F   C. F   D. T   E. T

This patient has a pulmonary stenosis with an atrial septal defect. The high right ventricular pressures with normal pulmonary artery pressure (systolic gradient of 43 mmHg) indicates pulmonary stenosis. A pulmonary gradient of up to 20 mmHg is not significant as there is a Venturi effect across the pulmonary valve, giving rise to a small gradient. The step-up in oxygen saturation in the right atrium is due to a left-to-right shunt or atrial septal defect.

5.   A. F   B. T   C. F   D. T   E. T

Infective endocarditis is usually caused by Gram-positive cocci. Acute bacterial endocarditis requires empiric antimicrobial treatment before culture report becomes available. *Staphylococcus aureus* and Gram-positive cocci are the most likely organisms. Subacute bacterial endocarditis is most often caused by streptococci. Endocarditis caused by *Streptococcus bovis* is associated with lower gastrointestinal neoplasms. Endocarditis involving the tricuspid or pulmonary valve is seen most frequently in parenteral drug abusers or in patients with intravascular catheters.

6.   A. F   B. T   C. T   D. F   E. F

Penicillin therapy results in cure in over 90% of patients with subacute bacterial endocarditis caused by streptococci. Penicillin plus an aminoglycoside are the treatment of choice for enterococcal endocarditis. *Staphylococcus aureus* endocarditis should be treated with cloxacillin, oxacillin or naficillin. In *Staphylococcus epidermidis* endocarditis cephalosporins should not be used to treat methicillin-resistant strains. In well-established bacterial endocarditis, therapy should be initiated despite blood cultures remaining negative. Treatment usually includes penicillin or ampicillin plus an aminoglycoside.

7.   A. T   B. T   C. T   D. T   E. T

Indications for surgery in infective endocarditis include: (1) positive blood cultures or relapse after several days of the best available antibiotic therapy indicates valve replacement; (2) fungal endocarditis refractory to medical therapy; (3) prosthetic valve with non-streptococcal endocarditis; (4) refractory heart failure; (5) development of a new aneurysm of the sinus of Valsalva; (6) drainage of a myocardial or valve ring abscess; (7) prosthetic valve dysfunction or dehiscence or myocardial invasion.

8. *Antimicrobial prophylaxis for bacterial endocarditis is indicated for*

A. previous coronary artery bypass graft.
B. mitral valve prolapse without mitral regurgitation.
C. cardiac pacemakers.
D. implantable defibrillators.
E. calcific aortic stenosis.

A........... B.......... C.......... D.......... E..........

9. *The following associations are correct.*

A. Pericarditis–ST elevation.
B. Myocarditis–ST elevation.
C. Acute aortic dissection–ST elevation.
D. Pneumothorax–acute QRS shift
E. Acute cholecystitis–inferior ST elevation.

A........... B.......... C.......... D.......... E..........

10. *Increased CK-MB relative to total creatine kinase (CK) is seen in*

A. rhabdomyolysis.
B. extensive muscle trauma.
C. polymyositis.
D. acute myocardial infarction.
E. vigorous exercise in marathon runners.

A........... B.......... C.......... D.......... E..........

11. *The following statements about lactate dehydrogenase (LDH) are correct.*

A. The LDH1 isoenzyme is specific for myocardial necrosis.
B. The diagnostic sensitivity of the LDH isoenzymes is reduced in haemolysis.
C. Measurement of plasma LDH isoenzymes is useful in the early diagnosis of acute myocardial infarction.
D. Measurement of plasma LDH is necessary in all individuals in whom acute myocardial infarction is suspected.
E. An LDH1: LDH2 ratio greater than 1.0 is consistent with acute myocardial infarction.

A........... B.......... C.......... D.......... E..........

8.   A. F   B. F   C. F   D. F   E. T

Antimicrobial prophylaxis for bacterial endocarditis is not indicated for previous coronary artery bypass graft, mitral valve prolapse without mitral regurgitation, cardiac pacemakers and implantable defibrillators. It is recommended in rheumatic valvular disease, most congenital heart lesions (except uncomplicated atrial septal defect of the secundum type), valvular aortic stenosis, prosthetic heart valve, previously documented infective endocarditis, calcified aortic stenosis and calcified mitral valve.

9.   A. T   B. T   C. T   D. T   E. T

All these conditions have ECG findings similar to that seen in acute myocardial infarction. ST elevation is a feature of pericarditis and myocarditis and such patients warrant diagnostic echocardiography. In acute aortic dissection there may be non-specific ST–T changes or ST elevation or depression. Further investigation in these patients includes chest computer axial tomography (CT) or magnetic resonance imaging (MRI), transoesophageal echocardiography and aortography. In pneumothorax, ECG findings include new poor progression of R waves in chest leads V1–V6 or an acute QRS shift; a chest X-ray is diagnostic. In acute cholecystitis, patients may have inferior ST elevation and further investigation includes abdominal ultrasound. Inferior ST elevation or ST shifts in chest leads V1–V3 may be seen in pulmonary embolism and a ventilation–perfusion scan is indicated when the diagnosis is suspected.

10.   A. F   B. F   C. T   D. T   E. T

High percentage of CK-MB to total CK is seen in acute myocardial infarction, polymyositis, muscular dystrophy, myopathies, vigorous exercise in trained athletes and patients with chronic renal insufficiency. Other causes of increased plasma CK-MB include myocarditis, pericarditis, myocardial contusion/blunt chest trauma, defibrillation or cardiac surgery. Additional sources of CK-MB include bronchogenic carcinoma. Low percentage of CK-MB relative to total CK is seen in rhabdomyolysis and extensive muscle trauma. Elevated levels of CK-MB may also be seen in hypothyroidism due to delayed clearance of the enzyme.

11.   A. T   B. T   C. F   D. F   E. T

LDH exists as five isoenzymes and is present in most body tissues but the LDH1 isoenzyme is relatively specific for myocardial necrosis. An LDH1:LDH2 ratio greater than 1.0 is consistent with acute myocardial infarction. LDH is detectable 12 h after onset of chest pain, peaks around 24–48 h and remains elevated for 10–15 days after onset of symptoms. The measurement of LDH is not essential in all suspected cases of myocardial infarction but is a valuable adjunct to CK determinations in patients presenting 24 h or more after onset of symptoms. The diagnostic sensitivity and specificity of LDH isoenzymes are reduced in the presence of blood dyscrasias such as megaloblastic anaemia and haemolysis, renal failure and solid tumours that induce elevation of LDH.

12. *Drugs used to treat a 30-year-old Afro-Caribbean man with a blood pressure of 130/ 100 mmHg include*

    A. atenolol.
    B. thiazide diuretics.
    C. captopril.
    D. amlodipine.
    E. labetolol.

    A........... B.......... C.......... D.......... E..........

13. *Withdrawal of beta blockers abruptly may precipitate*

    A. unstable angina.
    B. myocardial infarction.
    C. bronchial asthma.
    D. arrhythmias.
    E. sudden death.

    A........... B.......... C.......... D.......... E..........

14. *In a 53-year-old patient with inferior wall myocardial infarction, hypotension, elevated jugular venous pulsation, right third and fourth heart sounds and clear lung fields*

    A. right precordial ECG leads are usually normal.
    B. the cardiac index is increased.
    C. the right atrial pressure is decreased.
    D. intravenous fluids should be administered despite an elevated jugular venous pulsation.
    E. the right ventricle is devoid of infarction.

    A........... B.......... C.......... D.......... E..........

15. *A 55-year-old patient with myocardial infarction and ventricular ectopic beats (VEs) should be considered for treatment with lidocaine when the VEs*

    A. occur more frequently than $5\,min^{-1}$.
    B. lack an R–on–T phenomenon.
    C. occur in salvos of two or more.
    D. are associated with haemodynamic compromise.
    E. routinely in almost all patients with myocardial infarction.

    A........... B.......... C.......... D.......... E..........

16. *Accelerated idioventricular rhythm*

    A. occurs frequently in patients with coronary reperfusion.
    B. is a wide complex escape rhythm.
    C. occurs when the sinus rate slows below $60\,beats\,min^{-1}$.
    D. is usually accompanied by haemodynamic compromise.
    E. is usually treated with immediate defibrillation to prevent deterioration to ventricular fibrillation.

    A........... B.......... C.......... D.......... E..........

12. A. F   B. T   C. T   D. T   E. T

Black hypertensive patients tend to have a lower plasma renin activity, higher plasma volume and higher vascular resistance than white patients. Thus black patients tend to respond poorly to β-blockers but respond well to diuretics, alone or in combination with calcium channel blockers. One of the important mechanisms of action of β-blockers includes reducing plasma renin activity. Other drugs effective in black patients include angiotensin-converting enzyme (ACE) inhibitors and labetolol (the latter is an α and β blocker).

13. A. T   B. T   C. F   D. T   E. T

Infrequently, abrupt withdrawal of β-blockers may precipitate unstable angina, myocardial infarction, arrhythmias and even sudden death. Thus, when β-blockers have to be stopped suddenly, patients at a high risk for these complications must be monitored for sympathetic overactivity.

14. A. F   B. F   C. F   D. T   E. F

Inferior wall myocardial infarction, hypotension, elevated jugular venous pulsation, right third and fourth heart sounds and clear lung fields are recognised features of right ventricular infarction. Characteristic features include a decreased cardiac index, with normal or decreased left ventricular filling pressures and elevated right atrial pressures. Patients with hypotension and a decreased cardiac index often respond to intravenous fluids, although excessive fluid administration should be avoided. Patients with resistant hypotension (to intravenous fluids and dobutamine) should be treated with intra-aortic balloon counterpulsation.

15. A. T   B. F   C. T   D. T   E. F

Ventricular ectopic beats occur commonly following an acute myocardial infarction and should not be routinely treated. Treatment should be considered when they occur more frequently than 5 min^{-1}, occur in salvos of two or more, are associated with haemodynamic compromise or when the 'R-on-T' phenomenon occurs (i.e. the R wave of the ectopic beat falls on the T wave of a normal beat) as the latter can lead to ventricular fibrillation and death.

16. A. T   B. T   C. T   D. F   E. F

Accelerated idioventricular rhythm occurs frequently in patients with coronary reperfusion and less commonly in other patients with acute myocardial infarction. It is a wide complex escape rhythm that is associated with bradycardia. It is uncommonly associated with haemodynamic compromise and treatment is not required. It is self-limiting within 48 hours. Associated haemodynamic compromise indicates that the rhythm may deteriorate to ventricular tachycardia or fibrillation and treatment in such patients includes administration of atropine or overdrive pacing.

17.   *The following statements about myocardial infarction are correct.*

    A. The majority of transmural acute myocardial infarcts are caused by an occlusive intracoronary thrombus overlying an ulcerated or fissured stenotic plaque.

    B. Occlusion of a major coronary artery results in ischaemia throughout the anastomotic region supplied by that artery, most pronounced in the subendocardium.

    C. Although myocardial function becomes strikingly abnormal within 1 min after the onset of ischaemia, myocardial coagulation necrosis occurs only after 20–40 min of ischaemia.

    D. Occlusion of the left anterior descending coronary artery causes damage to the anterior wall of the left ventricle near the apex and anterior two-thirds of the interventricular septum.

    E. Thrombolytic therapy causes lysis of the thrombus and the underlying atherosclerotic plaque that initiated it.

    A...........   B..........   C..........   D..........   E..........

18.   *The following statements about myocardial infarction are correct.*

    A. Atrial infarction occurs in over two-thirds of patients with acute myocardial infarction.

    B. A stunned myocardium may not be capable of sustaining life.

    C. In about one-quarter of patients with myocardial infarction, the onset is entirely asymptomatic.

    D. Reperfusion injury causes stunned myocardium.

    E. Sudden cardiac death occurs in about one-fifth of patients after an infarct.

    A...........   B..........   C..........   D..........   E..........

19.   *Complications of myocardial infarction include*

    A. cardiac arrhythmias.

    B. left ventricular congestive failure.

    C. cardiogenic shock.

    D. rupture of the left ventricular free wall.

    E. thromboembolism.

    A...........   B..........   C..........   D..........   E..........

20.   *Hypertension*

    A. can be diagnosed on the basis of one measurement if it is accompanied by damage to the target organs.

    B. in an elderly individual with a palpable brachial artery that persists after cuff inflation excludes the possibility of pseudohypertension.

    C. is present when the average blood pressure is greater than 140 mmHg systolic and 90 mmHg diastolic.

    D. in patients with large arms is best measured with a small blood pressure cuff.

    E. is due to secondary causes in most patients.

    A...........   B..........   C..........   D..........   E..........

17.   A. T   B. T   C. T   D. T   E. F

At least 90% of transmural acute myocardial infarcts are caused by an occlusive intracoronary thrombus overlying an ulcerated or fissured stenotic plaque. Occlusion of a major coronary artery results in ischaemia throughout the anastomotic region supplied by that artery, most pronounced in the subendocardium. Although, myocardial function becomes strikingly abnormal within 1 min after the onset of ischaemia, myocardial coagulation necrosis occurs only after 20–40 min of ischaemia. Occlusion of the left anterior descending coronary artery causes damage to the anterior wall of the left ventricle near the apex and anterior two-thirds of the interventricular septum. The right coronary artery occlusion causes infarct of the inferior and posterior wall of the left ventricle, posterior one-third of the interventricular septum and posterior right ventricular free wall in most cases. Occlusion of the left circumflex coronary artery causes infarct of the lateral wall of the left ventricle. Thrombolytic therapy causes lysis of the thrombus occluding the coronary artery but insignificant changes take place in the underlying atherosclerotic plaque that initiated it.

18.   A. F   B. T   C. F   D. F   E. T

Atrial infarction occurs in less than 10% of patients with acute myocardial infarction, most often in conjunction with a large posterior left ventricular infarct. Reperfusion injury is cell death induced by reperfusion of myocytes that were still viable before reperfusion. Although most of the viable myocardium following reperfusion ultimately recovers, the function of these salvaged myocytes may be abnormal for days; this is known as stunned myocardium. Although normal function is ultimately recovered, stunned myocardium may not be capable of sustaining life. Sudden cardiac death occurs in about 20% of patients with acute myocardial infarction and occurs usually within 1–2 h after onset of symptoms. In about 10–15% of patients with myocardial infarction, the onset is entirely asymptomatic.

19.   A. T   B. T   C. T   D. T   E. T

Complications of acute myocardial infarction include cardiac arrhythmias, left ventricular congestive failure and mild-to-severe pulmonary oedema, cardiogenic shock, rupture of the left ventricular free wall, septum or papillary muscle and thromboembolism.

20.   A. T   B. F   C. T   D. F   E. F

Hypertension can be diagnosed on the basis of one measurement if it is accompanied by damage to the target organs including retina, brain, heart or kidneys or if greater than 210/120 mmHg. Three or more abnormal readings should be present, preferably over a period of several weeks, before treatment is begun. Hypertension is present when the average blood pressure is greater than 140 mmHg systolic and 90 mmHg diastolic. Blood pressure should be measured with a cuff of appropriate size; use of small cuffs results in inappropriately elevated blood pressure recordings. In most cases the cause of hypertension is not known and secondary hypertension comprises about 10% of cases.

21. *Ambulatory blood pressure recordings are useful in*

    A. suspected cases of 'white coat hypertension'.
    B. borderline elevated blood pressure recordings with target organ damage.
    C. the evaluation of resistance to drug therapy.
    D. labile hypertension.
    E. patients with postural hypotension.

    A.......... B.......... C.......... D.......... E..........

22. *A diagnosis of secondary hypertension should be considered when*

    A. the age of onset is less than 30 years.
    B. the hypertension is difficult to control after therapy has been initiated.
    C. stable hypertension becomes difficult to control.
    D. accelerated or malignant hypertension is present.
    E. there are signs of Cushing's syndrome.

    A.......... B.......... C.......... D.......... E..........

23. *Causes of secondary hypertension include*

    A. Shy–Drager syndrome.
    B. coarctation of aorta.
    C. Conn's syndrome.
    D. renal artery stenosis.
    E. phaeochromocytoma.

    A.......... B.......... C.......... D.......... E..........

24. *The following statements about the management of hypertension are correct.*

    A. Recent evidence has shown that life-long treatment is no longer required.
    B. Symptoms are a reliable gauge of treatment.
    C. The goal of treatment is to prevent damage to target organs.
    D. Isolated systolic hypertension does not require treatment.
    E. Blood pressure should be aggressively and rapidly reduced to prevent cerebral ischaemia.

    A.......... B.......... C.......... D.......... E..........

25. *In the following hypertensive patients the drugs of first choice are correct.*

    A. Young (less than 35 years) male hypertensive patients: β-blockers.
    B. Elderly hypertensive patients: β-blockers.
    C. In patients with congestive heart failure: β-blockers.
    D. With acute myocardial infarction: calcium channel blockers.
    E. Diabetic nephropathy with proteinuria: ACE inhibitors.

    A.......... B.......... C.......... D.......... E..........

21.   A. T   B. T   C. T   D. T   E. T

Ambulatory blood pressure recordings are useful in (1) suspected cases of 'white-coat hypertension' which is associated with the stress of visits to the doctor; (2) patients with borderline elevated blood pressure recordings or high normal readings with target organ damage; (3) the evaluation of resistance to drug therapy; (4) labile hypertension; and (5) patients with postural hypotension.

22.   A. T   B. T   C. T   D. T   E. T

A diagnosis of secondary hypertension should be considered when (1) the age of onset is less than 30 years or more than 60 years; (2) hypertension is difficult to control after therapy has been initiated; (3) stable hypertension becomes difficult to control; (4) accelerated or malignant hypertension is present; or (5) the signs of secondary causes are present.

23.   A. F   B. T   C. T   D. T   E. T

Less than 10% of hypertensive patients have a secondary cause and these include renal parenchymal and renovascular disease, coarctation of aorta, phaeochromocytoma, Conn's syndrome (primary hyperaldosteronism) and Cushing's syndrome. Shy–Drager syndrome is autonomic failure and is associated with postural hypotension.

24.   A. F   B. F   C. T   D. F   E. F

The goal of treatment in hypertension is to prevent damage to the target organs and the treatment is life-long. Isolated systolic hypertension with a systolic blood pressure greater than 160 mmHg should be treated to reduce the incidence of strokes and cardiac events. Blood pressure should not be aggressively and rapidly reduced to avoid cerebral ischaemia.

25.   A. F   B. F   C. F   D. F   E. T

In young (less than 35 years) male patients, although β-blockers are effective they may decrease serum high-density lipoprotein (HDL) levels, cause erectile dysfunction or retard physical and cardiac output by decreasing cardiac performance. In elderly hypertensive patients, diuretics are the drugs of first choice as they have been shown to reduce the incidence of stroke, fatal myocardial infarction and mortality. In patients with congestive heart failure, ACE inhibitors decrease mortality. Diuretics alone or in combination with calcium channel blockers are effective. In diabetic nephropathy with proteinuria, ACE inhibitors are used as first line as they reduce proteinuria and slow the loss of renal function independent of their antihypertensive effects. In patients with acute myocardial infarction, calcium channel blockers have to be used with caution as conflicting data exist on their adverse effects. ACE inhibitors, β-blockers and nitrates are useful in hypertensive patients with coronary artery disease.

26. *Side-effects of calcium channel blockers include*

A. impaired glucose tolerance.
B. elevated serum low-density lipoprotein (LDL) levels.
C. hyperkalaemia.
D. orthostatic hypotension.
E. lower leg oedema.

A.......... B.......... C.......... D.......... E..........

27. *The following statements about diuretics and their mechanisms of action are correct.*

A. Hydrochlorothiazide – blocks reabsorption in the thick ascending loop of Henle.
B. Bumetanide – blocks sodium reabsorption in the distal convoluted tubule.
C. Spironolactone – stimulates the action of aldosterone in the kidney.
D. Triamterene – inhibits the secretion of potassium ions in the distal tubule.
E. Frusemide blocks sodium reabsorption in the distal convoluted tubule.

A.......... B.......... C.......... D.......... E..........

28. *ACE inhibitors cause*

A. hypokalaemia.
B. hypercholesterolaemia.
C. hyperglycaemia.
D. hyperuricaemia.
E. hypercalcaemia.

A.......... B.......... C.......... D.......... E..........

29. *The use of intravenous antihypertensive agents is indicated in patients with*

A. intracranial haemorrhage.
B. aortic dissection.
C. rapidly progressive renal failure.
D. eclampsia.
E. accelerated malignant hypertension.

A.......... B.......... C.......... D.......... E..........

30. *Hypertension is associated with acute withdrawal of the following substances:*

A. alcohol.
B. cocaine.
C. narcotic analgesics.
D. clonidine
E. β-blockers.

A.......... B.......... C.......... D.......... E..........

26.   A. F   B. F   C. F   D. T   E. T

Calcium channel blockers do not have any significant effects on electrolytes, glucose tolerance or lipid levels. Verapamil may cause nausea, orthostatic hypotension, constipation, nausea and headache. Diltiazem may cause rash, nausea and headache. Nifedipine and other dihydropyridines may cause lower leg oedema, headache, flushing and skin rash.

27.   A. F   B. F   C. F   D. T   E. F

Hydrochlorothiazide blocks sodium reabsorption predominantly in the distal convoluted tubule. Loop diuretics such as frusemide, bumetanide and ethacrynic acid block reabsorption in the thick ascending loop of Henle. Spironolactone inhibits the action of aldosterone on the kidney. Triamterene and amiloride are potassium-sparing drugs that inhibit the secretion of potassium ions in the distal convoluted tubule.

28.   A. F   B. F   C. F   D. F   E. F

ACE inhibitors can reduce hypokalaemia, hypercholesterolaemia, hyperglycaemia and hyperkalaemia resulting from diuretic therapy; they are particularly effective when the plasma renin activity is high (e.g. renal crisis in scleroderma).

29.   A. T   B. T   C. T   D. T   E. T

Intravenous antihypertensive agents are indicated in patients with aortic dissection, eclampsia, rapidly progressive renal failure, intracranial haemorrhage and accelerated malignant hypertension.

30.   A. T   B. T   C. T   D. T   E. T

Hypertension is associated with the acute withdrawal of alcohol, cocaine, narcotic analgesics, clonidine and β-blockers.

31.   *The following are drugs of first choice for controlling blood pressure in the listed conditions.*

   A. Acute withdrawal syndrome caused by clonidine: β-adrenergic blockers.
   B. Hypertensive crisis associated with phaeochromocytoma: β-adrenergic blockers.
   C. Eclampsia: ACE inhibitors.
   D. Acute withdrawal syndrome caused by narcotic analgesic: clonidine.
   E. Hypertension associated with aortic dissection: sodium nitroprusside without β-blockers.

   A.......... B.......... C.......... D.......... E..........

32.   *Quinidine*

   A. is useful in suppressing both atrial and ventricular ectopic rhythms.
   B. acts predominantly by impeding sodium influx during phase 0 of the cardiac action potential.
   C. causes cinchonism.
   D. can increase serum digoxin two-fold with therapeutic doses.
   E. potentiates the effects of warfarin.

   A.......... B.......... C.......... D.......... E..........

33.   *Procainamide*

   A. is metabolised to N-acetylprocainamide, which is inert.
   B. is more effective than lidocaine in the acute termination of sustained ventricular tachycardia.
   C. causes a lupus-like syndrome.
   D. has β-adrenergic blocking effects.
   E. serum half-life may be significantly prolonged by cardiac failure.

   A.......... B.......... C.......... D.......... E..........

34.   *Lidocaine*

   A. is used as routine prophylaxis in acute myocardial infarction.
   B. is effective in preventing the recurrence of sustained life-threatening ventricular arrhythmias.
   C. is effective in the management of supraventricular arrhythmias.
   D. prolongs repolarisation time.
   E. causes negative inotropic effects even at low levels.

   A.......... B.......... C.......... D.......... E..........

31.   A. F   B. F   C. F   D. T   E. F

β-Blockers should not used in hypertension associated with phaeochromocytoma or clonidine withdrawal because unopposed α-adrenergic activity will be increased and may worsen the hypertension. The use of ACE inhibitors in pregnancy has been shown to increase perinatal morbidity or mortality. Clonidine is used to treat acute withdrawal syndrome caused by narcotic analgesics. Nitroprusside alone results in increased left ventricular wall pressure and the subsequent arterial shearing forces contribute to ongoing intimal dissection.

32.   A. T   B. T   C. T   D. T   E. T

Quinidine is useful in suppressing both atrial and ventricular ectopic rhythms. It is beneficial in preventing or terminating paroxysmal supraventricular tachycardia, preventing recurrent atrial fibrillation and converting atrial fibrillation. It acts predominantly by impeding sodium influx during phase 0 of the cardiac action potential. It causes cinchonism, which includes central nervous system (CNS) symptoms such as tinnitus, hearing deficits, visual disturbances, psychosis and delirium. Quinidine can increase ventricular rate by causing increased atriventricular node conduction by its vagolytic effect. Therefore, when quinidine is used in atrial tachyarrhythmias, atrioventricular node blocking drugs should be used before initiating quinidine therapy. It also causes hypotension and 'quinidine syncope', which is the result of recurrent episodes of torsades de pointes associated with QT prolongation. Severe left ventricular dysfunction, hypokalaemia and hypomagnesaemia all predispose patients to quinidine syncope. Therapeutic doses of quinidine can increase serum digoxin levels two-fold and potentiate the effects of warfarin.

33.   A. F   B. T   C. T   D. F   E. T

Procainamide acts on the fast sodium channel but its major metabolite, N-acetylprocainamide, can prolong repolarisation like other class III cardiac antiarrhythmics. It is more effective than lidocaine in the acute termination of sustained ventricular tachycardia, it's clinical utility is similar to quinidine and it has no β-blocking effects. Procainamide can cause a lupus-like syndrome, which produces a high titre of antinuclear antibodies but usually spares the kidneys. Its serum half-life is prolonged in cardiac failure or azotaemia.

34.   A. F   B. F   C. F   D. F   E. F

Lidocaine is useful in the management of ventricular tachyarrhythmias, particularly following a myocardial infarction, but is not used as routine prophylaxis in acute myocardial infarction. It acts on the fast sodium channels and intracardiac conduction and shortens repolarisation time. Lidocaine's negative inotropic effects occur only at high serum levels of the drug.

35. *β-Adrenergic blockers are useful in the management of*

   A. myocardial infarction.
   B. thyrotoxicosis.
   C. phaeochromocytoma.
   D. supraventricular arrhythmias
   E. neurocardiogenic syncope.

   A.......... B......... C.......... D.......... E..........

36. *Adverse effects of amiodarone therapy include*

   A. photosensitive skin rash.
   B. transient rise in hepatic transaminases.
   C. pulmonary fibrosis.
   D. corneal microdeposits.
   E. either hypothyroidism or hyperthyroidism.

   A.......... B......... C.......... D.......... E..........

37. *Adenosine*

   A. is contraindicated when re-entrant supraventricular tachycardia is present.
   B. is effective in converting atrial flutter to sinus rhythm.
   C. increases atrioventricular node conduction.
   D. has a serum half-life of 24 h.
   E. is more effective in patients who have ingested caffeine.

   A.......... B......... C.......... D.......... E..........

38. *Indications for digoxin treatment include*

   A. heart failure due to hypertrophic cardiomyopathy.
   B. Wolff–Parkinson–White syndrome.
   C. bidirectional ventricular tachycardia.
   D. atrial fibrillation.
   E. complete heart block.

   A.......... B......... C.......... D.......... E..........

35.   A. T   B. T   C. T   D. T   E. T

β-Blockers reduce both overall mortality and sudden death following acute myocardial infarction. They are useful in the management of sinus tachycardia, supraventricular tachycardias, atrial flutter and fibrillation by reducing the ventricular rate, particularly in the postoperative setting in cardiac surgical patients. β-Blockers are useful in the management of neurocardiogenic syncope and congenital long QT syndromes, in the treatment of excessive adrenergic states including thyrotoxicosis and phaeochromocytoma, and are used to control blood pressure, benign essential tremor and increased intraocular pressure.

36.   A. T   B. T   C. T   D. T   E. T

Amiodarone causes violaceous skin pigmentation in sun-exposed areas that is often distressing to the patient. The blue-grey pigmentation may not completely resolve on cessation of therapy. Almost all patients have corneal microdeposits on slit-lamp examination, although only a few have symptoms, which include halos around lights at night. Amiodarone can cause either hypothyroidism or hyperthyroidism and thyroid function should be monitored annually in these patients. It can cause an asymptomatic transient rise in hepatic transaminases and the drug should be discontinued when the level is twice the baseline or when there is a three-fold increase. It causes pulmonary symptoms and interstitial infiltrates and a decrease in diffusing capacity. Amiodarone also potentiates the effects of warfarin and increases digoxin and flecainide levels.

37.   A. F   B. F   C. F   D. F   E. F

Adenosine depresses atrioventricular node conduction, prolongs atrioventricular node refractoriness and also inhibits sinus node automaticity. It is effective in the treatment of re-entrant supraventricular tachycardia. It is not effective in converting atrial flutter, atrial fibrillation or ventricular tachycardia to sinus rhythm. Adenosine has a serum half-life of about 10 min, which is not affected by kidney or liver failure. Methylxanthines including caffeine and theophylline antagonise the effects of adenosine. Its side-effects include facial flushing, shortness of breath and chest pressure, all of which are transient.

38.   A. F   B. F   C. F   D. T   E. F

Digoxin treatment is contraindicated in hypertrophic cardiomyopathy as it increases outflow obstruction. In patients with Wolff–Parkinson–White syndrome, digitalis is contraindicated because blocking of the atrioventricular node may facilitate conduction by the accessory pathway, potentially resulting in ventricular fibrillation. Digitalis is useful to control the ventricular rate in atrial flutter or atrial fibrillation. Digitalis toxicity may result in cardiac arrhythmias including bidirectional ventricular tachycardia or complete heart block.

39. *Indications for permanent cardiac pacing include*

    A. complete atrioventricular block.
    B. sinus node dysfunction with symptomatic bradycardia.
    C. recurrent syncope provoked by carotid sinus stimulation.
    D. permanent second-degree atrioventricular block with bradycardia.
    E. second-degree atrioventricular block with bilateral bundle branch atrioventricular block.

    A..........   B..........   C..........   D..........   E..........

40. *The following statements are correct.*

    A. Familial hypercholesterolaemia is due to a defect in the LDL receptor.
    B. Familial combined hyperlipoproteinaemia is associated with increased risk of vascular disease.
    C. Lipaemia retinalis is characteristically absent in hyperchylomicronaemia.
    D. Hyperchylomicronaemia is associated with pancreatitis.
    E. β-Blockers may cause low HDL-cholesterol levels.

    A..........   B..........   C..........   D..........   E..........

41. *The following statements about the treatment of hyperlipidaemia are correct.*

    A. Palm oil is recommended due to its low content of saturated fat.
    B. *Trans*-fatty acids raise LDL-cholesterol levels.
    C. Intake of polyunsaturated fat should exceed 15% of the calories.
    D. Cardioselective β-adrenergic blockers are preferred over non-cardioselective ones.
    E. Postmenopausal women may benefit from hormone replacement therapy (HRT) as first-line therapy.

    A..........   B..........   C..........   D..........   E..........

42. *The following statements are correct.*

    A. Simvastatin lowers HDL-cholesterol levels.
    B. Nicotinic acid raises HDL-cholesterol levels.
    C. Gemfibrozil lowers triglyceride levels.
    D. Gemfibrozil lowers LDL-cholesterol levels.
    E. Bile acid resins lower LDL-cholesterol levels.

    A..........   B..........   C..........   D..........   E..........

39.   A. T   B. T   C. T   D. T   E. T

All of the above are indications for permanent cardiac pacing including bradyarrhythmias, asymptomatic second degree Mobitz-II heart block and complete heart block.

40.   A. T   B. T   C. F   D. T   E. T

Familial hypercholesterolaemia is an autosomal dominant disorder due to a defect in the LDL receptor. Familial combined hyperlipoproteinaemia is associated with increased risk of vascular disease. Lipaemia retinalis, pancreatitis, eruptive xanthomas and hepatosplenomegaly are all features of hyperchylomicronaemia. Anabolic steroids, β-blockers, smoking, obesity, lack of exercise and androgens may cause low HDL-cholesterol levels.

41.   A. F   B. T   C. F   D. T   E. T

Palm and coconut oil should be avoided due to their high content of saturated fat. *Trans*-fatty acids raise LDL-cholesterol and lower HDL-cholesterol levels. *Trans*-fatty acids are produced when liquid oils are hydrogenated to produce solid fats. Intake of polyunsaturated fat should not exceed 10% of the calories because high dietary intake of polyunsaturated fat will raise LDL-cholesterol and lower HDL-cholesterol. Thiazides and β-adrenergic blockers raise LDL-cholesterol and lower HDL-cholesterol and therefore cardioselective β-adrenergic blockers are preferred over non-cardioselective ones. Postmenopausal women may benefit from HRT as first-line therapy where the effect is predominantly due to oestrogens. The addition of progesterone (which is required for women who have a uterus) may blunt the beneficial effects of oestrogen on lipids.

42.   A. F   B. T   C. T   D. T   E. T

Simvastatin slightly raises HDL-cholesterol levels and lowers LDL-cholesterol levels. Nicotinic acid is a water-soluble vitamin that can lower very low density lipoprotein (VLDL) up to 40%, lower LDL-cholesterol by 15–30% and raise HDL-cholesterol by 10–30%. In patients with a low level of HDL-cholesterol and a high level of LDL-cholesterol, nicotinic acid is often preferred. Gemfibrozil is a fibric acid derivative that lowers VLDL and raises HDL-cholesterol and produces a reduction of LDL-cholesterol in patients with elevated levels. It is useful in patients with hypertriglyceridaemia and is used together with bile acid resins for the treatment of combined hyperlipidaemia.

43.   *The following statements about hydroxymethylglutaryl coenzyme (HMG-CoA) reductase inhibitors are correct.*

A. They inhibit the rate-limiting step in cholesterol biosynthesis.
B. They lower triglyceride levels.
C. They increase LDL receptors.
D. They decreases mortality from cardiovascular disease.
E. They should be avoided in active liver disease.

A........... B........... C........... D........... E...........

44.   *The following statements about valvular heart disease are correct.*

A. If severe mitral disease is identified prior to pregnancy, valvotomy should be carried out before conception.
B. Pregnant women with mitral stenosis should be treated surgically even when asymptomatic.
C. Mitral regurgitation is usually poorly tolerated during pregnancy.
D. Aortic stenosis is a contraindication for pregnancy unless the lesion is corrected.
E. In patients with prosthetic valves, antibiotic prophylaxis against genitourinary organisms is mandatory during the peripartum period.

A........... B........... C........... D........... E...........

45.   *The following statements about cardiovascular disease in pregnancy are correct.*

A. Patients with Marfan's syndrome and dilated aortic root should avoid pregnancy.
B. In Eisenmenger's syndrome both maternal and fetal mortality are high.
C. Maternal atrial septal defect is associated with increased risk of fetal loss.
D. Hypertrophic cardiomyopathy is generally tolerated poorly in pregnancy.
E. Subsequent pregnancies should be avoided in patients with peripartum cardiomyopathy.

A........... B........... C........... D........... E...........

43.   A. T   B. F   C. T   D. T   E. T

HMG-CoA reductase inhibitors, which include lovastatin, simvastatin, pravastatin and fluvastatin, inhibit the rate-limiting step in cholesterol biosynthesis, causing a decrease in intracellular cholesterol and consequently an increase in LDL receptors. The Scandinavian Simvastatin Survival Study (4S) showed that simvastatin improves survival in patients with coronary artery disease; the West of Scotland Study showed that pravastatin prevents coronary artery disease in men with hypercholesterolaemia. These agents should be avoided in active liver disease as they can cause elevation of liver function tests and liver damage; thus liver function should be monitored in patients on therapy. In combination with gemfibrozil, erythromycin, niacin or cyclosporin, lovastatin has been shown to increase CK levels and increase the risk of myopathy and rhabdomyolysis.

44.   A. T   B. F   C. F   D. T   E. T

If severe mitral disease is identified prior to pregnancy, valvotomy should be carried out before conception. Pregnant women with mitral stenosis should not be treated surgically when asymptomatic. Mitral regurgitation is usually well tolerated during pregnancy. Aortic stenosis is a contraindication for pregnancy unless the lesion is corrected. In patients with prosthetic valves, antibiotic prophylaxis against genitourinary organisms is mandatory during the peripartum period.

45.   A. T   B. T   C. T   D. F   E. T

In Marfan's syndrome, pregnancy should be avoided as the risk of aortic dissection and rupture during pregnancy is increased when the diameter of the aortic root exceeds 40 mm. In Eisenmenger's syndrome, both fetal and maternal mortality are high, the latter increasing with the severity of the right-to-left shunt. Pulmonary hypertension is a contraindication during pregnancy. Patients with hypertrophic cardiomyopathy generally tolerate pregnancy well as the hypervolaemia is associated with a reduction in the pressure gradient in the ventricle. Atrial septal defect is well tolerated during pregnancy when not complicated by pulmonary hypertension, but the risk of fetal loss is increased. In peripartum cardiomyopathy, both infant and maternal mortality is high. About one-third show functional recovery, one-third have persistently impaired left ventricular dysfunction and the remaining one-third die. Subsequent pregnancies should be avoided.

46. *A 28-year-old woman with a diastolic blood pressure greater than 100 mmHg who is 18 weeks pregnant can be treated with the following drugs:*

 A. propranolol.
 B. nifedipine.
 C. captopril.
 D. methyldopa.
 E. hydrochlorothiazide.

 A............   B..........   C..........   D..........   E..........

47. *A 22-year-old pregnant women was diagnosed as having pre-eclampsia by her obstetrician because of the following features.*

 A. generalised seizures.
 B. hypertension.
 C. proteinuria.
 D. generalised oedema.
 E. abnormal liver function tests.

 A............   B..........   C..........   D..........   E..........

48. *The following are physiological changes in pregnancy.*

 A. Systemic vascular resistance is increased.
 B. The rise in cardiac output exceeds the increase in oxygen consumption.
 C. Blood pressure usually falls during the second trimester.
 D. Glomerular filtration rate (GFR) falls.
 E. A modest rise in blood pressure may occur in the last month of normal pregnancy.

 A............   B..........   C..........   D..........   E..........

46.   A. F   B. F   C. F   D. T   E. F

Chronic hypertension is defined as a blood pressure of greater than 140/90 mmHg before the twentieth week of pregnancy. Treatment is indicated when diastolic blood pressure is greater than 100 mmHg. α-Methyldopa is recommended as first-line treatment because of proven safety. An alternative agent is hydralazine, which can also be used parenterally. Propranolol and other β-blockers should be avoided because uterine contractility may increase and in the fetus and neonate they may cause bradycardia, intrauterine growth retardation, hyperbilirubinaemia, hypoglycaemia and delayed respiration. However, there are several studies showing the safety of labetolol (α + β blocker) in pregnancy. Calcium channel blockers including nifedipine should be avoided because they decrease uterine contractility and when combined with β-blockers cause high rates of Caesarean section, premature delivery and small-for-date infants. ACE inhibitors increase perinatal morbidity and mortality. Thiazide diuretics should be avoided because they decrease uterine blood flow and cause neonatal jaundice, hyponatraemia and thrombocytopenia.

47.   A. F   B. T   C. T   D. T   E. T

Pre-eclampsia is a condition defined by the presence of pregnancy, hypertension, proteinuria and generalised oedema. Other features include abnormal liver function tests and coagulation abnormalities. The presence of generalised seizures in addition to these abnormalities defines eclampsia. If a patient is suspected of having pre-eclampsia or eclampsia she should be referred to an obstetrician specialising in high-risk pregnancy. In these patients diazoxide may inhibit uterine contractions and trimetaphan can cause meconium ileus.

48.   A. F   B. T   C. T   D. F   E. T

Pregnancy is associated with a reduction in systemic vascular resistance. In the second trimester blood pressure falls, despite an increase in stroke volume and heart rate and a 40% increase in cardiac output. The rise in cardiac output usually exceeds the increase in oxygen consumption. A modest rise in blood pressure in the last month of pregnancy is normal; however, an increase in systolic blood pressure of 30 mmHg or diastolic pressure of 15 mmHg is pathological and merits treatment because of the increased risk of fetal growth retardation, mortality and maternal complications (pre-eclampsia). An increase in GFR is normal during pregnancy due to a rise in renal plasma flow; this is not accompanied by a rise in glomerular pressure. When the kidney is diseased any rise in GFR is accompanied by a rise in glomerular pressure, resulting in increased proteinuria and worsening of the underlying condition.

49.   *The following statements about the management of pre-eclampsia are correct.*

   A. Hospitalisation is indicated.
   B. The definitive treatment is delivery of the conceptus.
   C. ACE inhibitors are drugs of first choice to control elevated systemic blood
      pressures.
   D. Hydralazine is contraindicated.
   E. Intravenous magnesium sulphate is used to reduce blood pressure.

   A........... B.......... C.......... D.......... E..........

50.   *The following statements about the management of heart failure are correct.*

   A. Enalapril improves survival rates in mild to moderate heart failure.
   B. Hydralazine–isosorbide nitrate combination is superior to enalapril.
   C. Enalapril improves survival in patients with asymptomatic left ventricular
      dysfunction.
   D. Digoxin improves survival in patients with heart failure.
   E. Enalapril is particularly useful in those with underlying bilateral renal
      artery stenosis.

   A........... B.......... C.......... D.......... E..........

51.   *The following associations are correct.*

   A. Aortic stenosis–early diastolic murmur.
   B. Mitral stenosis–pansystolic murmur.
   C. Tricuspid stenosis–mid-diastolic murmur.
   D. Aortic regurgitation–early diastolic murmur.
   E. Mitral regurgitation–mid-diastolic murmur.

   A........... B.......... C.......... D.......... E..........

52.   *Recognised causes of aortic regurgitation include*

   A. systemic hypertension.
   B. ankylosing spondylitis.
   C. Marfan's syndrome.
   D. rheumatic fever.
   E. syphilis.

   A........... B.......... C.......... D.......... E..........

49.   A. T   B. T   C. F   D. F   E. T

Once a diagnosis of pre-eclampsia is made the patient should be hospitalised as she may rapidly deteriorate to eclampsia (manifested by convulsions). The definitive treatment of pre-eclampsia is the delivery of the fetus and should be done promptly, unless the fetus is immature. When the fetus is immature, patients should be treated conservatively with bed rest, restriction of salt (sodium less than $2\,g/day^{-1}$) and antihypertensive agents (β-blockers, calcium channel blockers, hydralazine and central sympatholytics). ACE inhibitors are contraindicated in pregnancy as they increase the risk of fetal loss. Intravenous magnesium sulphate reduces blood pressure and is said to increase the synthesis of prostacyclin (PGI_2), a vasodilating prostaglandin produced by endothelial cells.

50.   A. T   B. F   C. F   D. F   E. F

The SOLVD (Study of Left Ventricular Dysfunction) 'treatment' wing showed that enalapril improves survival rates in mild to moderate heart failure compared with placebo. The 'prevention' wing of this study showed that enalapril had no prognostic benefit in patients with asymptomatic left ventricular dysfunction (i.e. ejection fraction lower than 35%). However, these patients were less likely to progress to heart failure or to require hospital admissions. ACE inhibitors including enalapril should be avoided in patients with bilateral renal stenosis as they may precipitate acute renal failure. The recent DIG (Digoxin Investigation Group) trial showed that digoxin does not reduce overall mortality but reduces the number of hospital admissions (both overall and for worsening heart failure).

51.   A. F   B. F   C. T   D. T   E. F

The murmurs of aortic stenosis, mitral stenosis, tricuspid stenosis, aortic regurgitation and mitral regurgitation are ejection systolic, mid-diastolic, early diastolic and pansystolic respectively.

52.   A. T   B. T   C. T   D. T   E. T

Causes of chronic aortic regurgitation include rheumatic fever, hypertension, bacterial endocarditis, idiopathic dilatation of the aortic root and annulus, syphilis, Marfan's syndrome, rheumatoid arthritis, cystic medial necrosis, ankylosing spondylitis and bicuspid aortic valve. Causes of acute aortic regurgitation include infective endocarditis, aortic dissection, trauma, failure of aortic prosthetic valve and rupture of the sinus of Valsalva.

53. *The following statements are correct.*

A. Balloon valvuloplasty is preferred to valve replacement in the management of aortic stenosis.
B. Long-term vasodilator therapy with nifedipine reduces or delays the need for aortic valve replacement in asymptomatic patients with severe aortic regurgitation.
C. Patients with aortic regurgitation in whom left ventricular dysfunction developed when treated with nifedipine respond favourably to valve replacement in terms of survival and normalisation of ejection fraction.
D. Patients with mitral stenosis usually become symptomatic in the second trimester of pregnancy.
E. In atrial septal defect, large flow murmurs across the tricuspid valve can cause mid-diastolic murmurs.

A.......... B.......... C.......... D.......... E..........

54. *The following statements are correct.*

A. The third heart sound is due to vigorous contraction of the atria (atrial systole).
B. The fourth heart sound is due to rapid ventricular filling in early diastole.
C. In patients with mitral regurgitation, a third heart sound usually indicates the presence of systolic dysfunction and raised filling pressure.
D. In aortic stenosis, third heart sounds do not necessarily reflect ventricular systolic dysfunction or increased filling pressure.
E. The fourth heart sound denotes heart failure.

A.......... B.......... C.......... D.......... E..........

55. *Recognised causes of tricuspid regurgitation include*

A. rheumatic fever.
B. blunt trauma to heart.
C. Ebstein's anomaly.
D. carcinoid syndrome.
E. endomyocardial fibrosis.

A.......... B.......... C.......... D.......... E..........

56. *Widely split second sound occurs in*

A. aortic stenosis.
B. pulmonary stenosis.
C. right bundle branch block.
D. atrial septal defect.
E. left bundle branch block.

A.......... B.......... C.......... D.......... E..........

53.   A. F   B. T   C. T   D. T   E. T

Balloon valvuloplasty should be limited to moribund patients requiring emergency intervention or those with a very poor life expectation due to other pathology. In one study, although in-hospital mortality was similar to that following conventional surgical valve replacement, there were more deaths in the valvuloplasty group in the subsequent follow-up period. Long-term vasodilator therapy with nifedipine reduces or delays the need for aortic valve replacement in asymptomatic patients with severe aortic regurgitation. Patients with aortic regurgitation in whom left ventricular dysfunction developed when treated with nifedipine respond favourably to valve replacement in terms of survival and normalisation of ejection fraction. Patients with mitral stenosis usually become symptomatic in the second trimester of pregnancy. In atrial septal defect, large flow murmurs across the tricuspid valve can cause mid-diastolic murmurs.

54.   A. F   B. F   C. F   D. F   E. F

The third heart sound is due to rapid ventricular filling in early diastole. The fourth heart sound is due to vigorous contraction of the atria (atrial systole) and hence is towards the end of diastole. In patients with mitral stenosis, third heart sounds are common but do not necessarily reflect ventricular systolic dysfunction or increased filling pressure. In aortic stenosis, third heart sounds are uncommon but usually indicate the presence of systolic dysfunction and raised filling pressure. The fourth heart sound does not denote heart failure, unlike the S3 gallop.

55.   A. T   B. T   C. T   D. T   E. T

Causes of tricuspid regurgitation include right heart bacterial endocarditis in intravenous drug abusers, carcinoid syndrome, Ebstein's anomaly, endomyocardial fibrosis, infarction of the right ventricular papillary muscles, tricuspid valve prolapse, blunt trauma to the heart and rheumatic fever.

56.   A. F   B. T   C. T   D. T   E. F

Abnormally widely split second sound occurs in atrial septal defect, ventricular septal defect, pulmonary regurgitation (due to increased right ventricular volume), pulmonary stenosis (due to increased right ventricular pressure), right bundle branch block (due to right ventricular conduction delay) and in mitral regurgitation and ventricular septal defect (due to premature left ventricular emptying). In left bundle branch block and aortic stenosis the second sound is narrowly split or has a reverse split.

57. *The following statements are correct.*

A. Intravenous heparin decreases the incidence of myocardial infarction in patients with unstable angina.
B. Prinzmetal's angina is associated with ST segment elevation.
C. Therapy for silent ischaemia is similar to that associated with symptoms.
D. Argatroban reduces mortality in unstable angina.
E. Non-Q wave myocardial infarcts are usually transmural infarcts.

A............   B..........   C..........   D..........   E..........

58. *A 60-year-old woman treated for 10 years for atrial fibrillation presented with nausea and vomiting. ECG showed a bidirectional ventricular tachycardia and electrolytes revealed hyperkalaemia.*

A. The nausea and vomiting is due to digitalis toxicity.
B. Life-threatening digoxin arrhythmias respond to Fab fragments of anti-digitalis antibody.
C. The hyperkalaemia is due to stimulation of the sodium–potassium ATPase pump.
D. Haemodialysis is helpful in such cases.
E. Intravenous calcium helps to reverse the arrhythmia.

A............   B..........   C..........   D..........   E..........

57.   A. T   B. T   C. T   D. T   E. F

Intravenous heparin decreases the incidence of myocardial infarction in patients with unstable angina. Prinzmetal's angina is characterised by episodes of chest pain occurring at rest associated with ST segment elevation due to coronary artery spasm. Silent ischaemia is defined as objective evidence of myocardial ischaemia in the absence of angina or anginal equivalents; the therapy for silent ischaemia is similar to that associated with symptoms. The PRISM trial showed that argatroban reduces mortality in unstable angina. Q wave myocardial infarcts are transmural infarcts.

58.   A. T   B. T   C. F   D. F   E. F

This patient has digitalis toxicity. The presence of nausea, vomiting and bidirectional ventricular tachycardia indicate digitalis toxicity. The hyperkalaemia is due to inhibition of the cellular sodium–potassium ATPase, which normally maintains the intracellular to extracellular concentration gradient for sodium and potassium. When life-threatening hypotension or arrhythmias occur, intravenous digoxin-immune Fab fragments should be given. Calcium increases the toxicity of digitalis and should be avoided. Haemodialysis and haemoperfusion are of no benefit in digitalis overdose.

2 METABOLISM AND ENDOCRINOLOGY

59. *A 33-year-old presented with excessive sweating, joint pain and difficulty in vision. Serum calcium was 2.6 mmol l^{-1}, urine calcium excretion 9.7 mmol day^{-1}, serum phosphate 1.8 mmol l^{-1}, alkaline phosphatase 102 IUL^{-1} and creatinine clearance 141 ml min^{-1}. The following investigations will be done to manage the patient:*

A. CT scan of pituitary fossa.
B. growth hormone levels after oral glucose.
C. static and dynamic tests of pituitary function.
D. renal artery angiogram.
E. plasma insulin-like growth factor (IGF) levels.

A............   B..........   C..........   D..........   E..........

60. *A 37-year-old woman had a plasma thyroxine level of 35.2 nmol l^{-1}, fasting plasma thyroid-stimulating hormone (TSH) was not detected. Following intravenous thyrotrophin-releasing hormone (TRH), plasma TSH was 10 times above control values. Recognised clinical features include*

A. myxoedema.
B. a history of post-partum haemorrhage.
C. absence of axillary hair.
D. atrophied breasts.
E. hyperpigmentation.

A............   B..........   C..........   D..........   E..........

61. *A girl aged 3 years with long-standing constipation has an abnormal facies and is on the tenth percentile for weight and on the third percentile for height. Investigations reveal a haemoglobin of 13 g dl^{-1}, serum calcium of 1.6 mmol l^{-1}, serum phosphate of 3 mmol l^{-1} and plasma creatinine of 46 µmol l^{-1}. The following are correct.*

A. This girl has hyperparathyroidism.
B. Parathormone levels will be appropriate to the calcium levels.
C. There is shortening of the fourth and fifth metacarpals.
D. There is end-organ resistance to parathormone.
E. The patient has hypopituitarism.

A............   B..........   C..........   D..........   E..........

59.   A. T   B. T   C. T   D. F   E. T

This patient has acromegaly and investigations to confirm the diagnosis include CT scan of pituitary fossa, formal perimetry, growth hormone levels after oral glucose, static and dynamic tests of pituitary function, triple stimulation test if hypopituitarism is suspected and plasma IFG levels (allows assessment of the efficacy of initial therapy and in the post-therapeutic approach).

60.   A. F   B. T   C. T   D. T   E. F

This patient has secondary hypothyroidism due to hypopituitarism. Recognised manifestations include postural hypotension, pale soft skin with paucity of axillary and pubic hair, and atrophy of breasts. The patient may give a history of amenorrhoea preceded by postpartum pituitary necrosis (known as Sheehan's syndrome). In general in hypopituitarism, growth hormone, follicle stimulating hormone (FSH) and luteinising hormone (LH) secretions become deficient early followed by TSH and adrenocorticotrophic hormone (ACTH). Last of all, antidiuretic hormone secretions diminish and fail.

61.   A. F   B. T   C. T   D. T   E. F

This patient has pseudohypoparathyroidism where the facies are rounded and flat. There is shortening of the fourth and fifth metacarpals. Parathormone levels will be appropriate to the calcium levels but there is end-organ resistance to parathormone, which may be partial or complete.

62. *An 80-year-old man who lives alone complained of increasing back and pelvic pain for 2 years. Investigations revealed a creatinine clearance of $70 \, ml \, min^{-1}$, serum calcium of $2 \, mmol \, l^{-1}$, serum inorganic phosphate of $0.6 \, mmol \, l^{-1}$, serum urate of $0.4 \, mmol \, l^{-1}$, alkaline phosphatase of $130 \, IU \, l^{-1}$ and urine calcium of $5.1 \, mmol \, l^{-1}$.*

    A. All the above changes can be explained by vitamin A intoxication.
    B. Renal function may be considered normal for the age.
    C. The calcium levels can be explained by hyperparathyroidism.
    D. Vitamin D should not be administered.
    E. X-rays of pelvis will show Looser's zones.

    A........... B.......... C.......... D.......... E..........

63. *A 30-year-old male with known complete failure of the anterior pituitary was on replacement cortisol and thyroxine therapy. Following an initial period of improvement he had nocturia. He underwent a fluid deprivation test. Baseline values were weight 73 kg, urine osmolarity $335 \, mmol \, l^{-1}$ and plasma osmolarity $295 \, mmol \, l^{-1}$. After withholding fluids for 8 h his weight was 68.9 kg, urine osmolarity $240 \, mmol \, l^{-1}$ and plasma osmolarity $303 \, mmol \, l^{-1}$. The following statements are correct.*

    A. These findings indicate the presence of hysterical polydipsia.
    B. The administration of cortisol unmasked his deficiency.
    C. Antidiuretic hormone has no effect in this patient.
    D. The cortisol should be stopped to reduce his symptoms.
    E. These symptoms can be explained by renal resistance to antidiuretic hormone.

    A........... B.......... C.......... D.......... E..........

64. *Insulin is necessary for*

    A. transmembrane transport of glucose.
    B. glycogen formation in the liver.
    C. conversion of glucose to triglycerides.
    D. nucleic acid synthesis.
    E. protein synthesis.

    A........... B.......... C.......... D.......... E..........

65. *Postulated mechanisms for long-standing complications of diabetes mellitus include*

    A. accumulation of irreversible advanced glycosylation end-products (AGEs) in the vessel wall.
    B. increased myoinositol content in Schwann cells.
    C. accumulation of sorbitol.
    D. inhibition of aldol reductase.
    E. decreased sodium–potassium ATPase activity.

    A........... B.......... C.......... D.......... E..........

62. A. F   B. T   C. F   D. F   E. T

This man has an elevated alkaline phosphatase and a low serum calcium level that is probably due to osteomalacia. The X-rays of the bone may show pseudofractures or Looser's zones. Management includes vitamin D. Renal function in this patient can be considered normal for his age.

63. A. F   B. T   C. F   D. F   E. F

This patient has diabetes insipidus, which is demonstrated by the inability of the urine to concentrate following fluid deprivation. A normal response to an 8-h fluid deprivation is a 0.5-kg loss of body weight and a rise in urine osmolarity to $700-1000 \, \text{mmol} \, l^{-1}$. Nocturia developed because cortisol increases the ability to excrete water and thus unmasks the posterior pituitary failure he had in addition to anterior pituitary failure.

64. A. T   B. T   C. T   D. T   E. T

The prime metabolic function of insulin is to increase glucose transport into certain cells, particularly striated muscle cells, cardiac muscle cells, fibroblasts and fats cells, which collectively constitute about two-thirds of the entire body weight. One of the important early effects of insulin action involves the translocation of glucose transport protein units (GLUTs) from the Golgi apparatus to the plasma membrane thus facilitating cellular uptake of glucose. GLUT-4, present in muscle and adipose tissue, is the major insulin-regulatable transporter. Insulin is also necessary for transmembrane transport of amino acids, glycogen formation in the liver and skeletal muscles, glucose conversion to triglycerides, nucleic acid synthesis and protein synthesis.

65. A. T   B. F   C. T   D. F   E. T

Glucose forms chemically reversible glycosylation products with protein (named Schiff bases) that may rearrange to form more stable Amadori-type early glycosylation products which are also chemically reversible. Rather than dissociating, the early glycosylation products on collagen and other long-lived proteins in interstitial tissues and blood vessel walls undergo a series of slow chemical rearrangements to form irreversible AGEs, which accumulate over the lifetime of the vessel wall. AGEs accumulate at a faster rate in the arteries and plasma of diabetic patients compared with control subjects and AGE peptide serum levels correlate with the severity of nephropathy. Hyperglycaemia leads to increased intracellular glucose in some tissues (nerve, lens, kidney and blood vessels) which is then metabolised to sorbitol by aldose reductase and eventually to fructose. The excess of sorbitol and fructose causes increased intracellular osmolarity and influx of water and osmotic cell injury. The accumulation of sorbitol is associated with a decrease of myoinositol content, resulting in decreased phosphoinositide metabolism, diacylglycerol, protein kinase C and sodium–potassium ATPase activity. This mechanism has been implicated in damage to Schwann cells and pericytes of retinal capillaries, causing peripheral neuropathy and retinal microaneurysms respectively. In the lens, osmotically imbibed water causes swelling and opacity (i.e. cataracts).

66.   *The following statements about glucose metabolism are correct.*

A. Patients with impaired glucose tolerance have an increased risk of development of macrovascular complications without manifesting overt diabetes mellitus.
B. In gestational diabetes, glucose tolerance usually reverts to normal following delivery.
C. Individuals with gestational diabetes have increased risk of development of diabetes mellitus later in life.
D. Thiazide diuretics cause reversible inhibition of insulin secretion.
E. Glucocorticoids may promote transient hyperglycaemia among patients without established diabetes mellitus.

A..........   B..........   C..........   D..........   E..........

67.   *The following statements about monitoring therapy in diabetes mellitus are correct.*

A. Falsely high plasma glucose values may occur as a result of glycolysis in collection tubes.
B. Urine glucose measured using glucose oxidase reagent strips correlates well with blood glucose levels.
C. Glycated haemoglobin (haemoglobin A_{1c}) assays correlate with mean blood glucose levels over 2–3 months preceding measurement.
D. Urine ketone measurement is a sensitive method of detecting ketones in the blood.
E. Capillary blood glucose measurement allows rapid determination of the glucose level in blood.

A..........   B..........   C..........   D..........   E..........

68.   *The following statements about dietary therapy in diabetes are correct.*

A. Complex carbohydrates should be avoided.
B. Proteins should not be limited in diabetic nephropathy.
C. Guar gum aids control of glucose.
D. Alcohol should be avoided in those with neuropathy.
E. Alcohol affects sulphonylurea metabolism.

A..........   B..........   C..........   D..........   E..........

66.   A. T   B. T   C. T   D. T   E. T

Patients with impaired glucose tolerance have an increased risk of development of macrovascular complications (stroke, myocardial infarction) without manifesting overt diabetes mellitus. In gestational diabetes, glucose tolerance usually reverts to normal following delivery. Individuals with gestational diabetes have increased risk of development of diabetes mellitus and impaired glucose tolerance later in life. Thiazide diuretics, phenytoin and diazoxide cause reversible inhibition of insulin secretion. Glucocorticoids, oestrogens, nicotinic acid and sympathomimetic drugs may promote transient hyperglycaemia among patients without established diabetes mellitus.

67.   A. F   B. F   C. T   D. T   E. T

Falsely low plasma glucose values may occur as a result of glycolysis in collection tubes; these can be minimised by the use of inhibitors of glycolysis. Urine glucose measured using glucose oxidase reagent strips correlates poorly with blood glucose levels. The excretion of glucose and water influence the measurement of urine glucose and hence glucose oxidase reagent strips are a semi-quantitative measurement. Urine assays cannot detect hypoglycaemia. Glycated haemoglobin (haemoglobin A_{1c}) assays correlate with mean blood glucose levels over 2–3 months preceding measurement as this occurs during the life span of red blood cells. In uraemia and haemolytic anaemia when red blood cell survival is reduced, haemoglobin A_{1c} levels may provide an underestimation of chronic hyperglycaemia. Haemoglobin A_{1c} should be measured at 2–3 monthly intervals in patients to validate the self-monitoring of blood glucose. Urine ketone measurement is a sensitive method of detecting ketones in the blood but urine ketones are of only limited utility in following therapy. Serial measurements of serum ketones are not helpful, because in diabetic ketoacidosis β-hydroxybutyrate is the most prevalent ketone and this is not detected by the nitroprusside reaction. Unless lactic acidosis is present, anion gap is a more reliable parameter of ketoacidosis. Capillary blood glucose measurement allows rapid determination of the glucose level in blood.

68.   A. F   B. F   C. T   D. T   E. T

Complex carbohydrates are the preferred source of energy in diabetic patients, whereas the intake of refined sugars should be avoided. Limitation of protein intake may be required in diabetic nephropathy. Fibre-containing foods, including guar gum, beans and legumes, aid control of glucose. Alcohol should be avoided in those with neuropathy. Alcohol affects sulphonylurea metabolism and may contribute to the development of lactic acidosis induced by sulphonylureas. Alcohol also inhibits liver gluconeogenesis and may exacerbate hypoglycaemia in patients on insulin or oral hypoglycaemic drugs.

69. *Recognised causes of diabetes mellitus include*

A. haemochromatosis.
B. Cushing's syndrome.
C. acromegaly.
D. pancreatectomy.
E. pentamidine isethionate.

A............   B..........   C..........   D..........   E..........

70. *The following statements about the management of diabetic ketoacidosis are correct.*

A. Bolus infusion of bicarbonate therapy should be routinely administered to prevent hyperchloraemia seen with administration of sodium chloride solutions.
B. Potassium replacement should be avoided to prevent intracellular hyperkalaemia.
C. Intravenous dextrose is administered when blood glucose falls to $200–300\,\mathrm{mg\,dl}^{-1}$ despite the presence of ketonuria and ketoacidosis.
D. Insulin treatment promotes elevation of plasma phosphate levels.
E. Intramuscular insulin is preferred in hypotensive patients.

A............   B..........   C..........   D..........   E..........

71. *Complications of diabetic ketoacidosis include*

A. hyperosmolar coma.
B. lactic acidosis.
C. stroke.
D. cerebral oedema.
E. myocardial infarction.

A............   B..........   C..........   D..........   E..........

72. *The following statements about the management of non-insulin-dependent diabetes mellitus (NIDDM) are correct.*

A. Sulphonylureas are particularly useful in pregnant adults.
B. Metformin may be particularly useful in patients with hyperlipidaemia.
C. Chlorpropamide is useful in alcoholic patients.
D. Metformin should be avoided in obese individuals.
E. Combined therapy with sulphonylurea and metformin may be used as an alternative therapy to insulin.

A............   B..........   C..........   D..........   E..........

69.   A. T   B. T   C. T   D. T   E. T

Haemochromatosis, Cushing's syndrome, acromegaly, pancreatectomy and cystic fibrosis are all recognised causes of secondary diabetes mellitus. Pentamidine isethionate and streptozotocin cause diabetes by the destruction of the insulin-producing β cells of the pancreas.

70.   A. F   B. F   C. T   D. F   E. F

Bolus infusion of bicarbonate therapy should be avoided unless the patient requires emergency resuscitation. In diabetic ketoacidosis, bicarbonate therapy is considered when the arterial pH is below 7.1, in severe hyperkalaemia or when the patient is in shock or coma. Sodium bicarbonate may be used in maintenance intravenous fluids regardless of the specific indication for bicarbonate therapy in order to reduce the hyperchloraemia seen with administration of sodium chloride solutions. Potassium replacement is essential in diabetic ketoacidosis, although hyperkalaemia is often observed initially because patients with diabetic ketoacidosis are usually potassium depleted and insulin therapy can induce life-threatening hyperkalaemia. Although insulin lowers blood glucose, the resolution of ketone production and acidosis is the therapeutic objective. Intravenous dextrose therapy is necessary because the fall in blood glucose with insulin therapy is usually more rapid than the resolution of ketoacidosis. Insulin treatment causes reduction of plasma phosphate levels by enhancing cellular uptake of phosphate. Intramuscular insulin should be avoided in hypotensive patients because absorption is unpredictable.

71.   A. F   B. T   C. T   D. T   E. T

Complications of diabetic ketoacidosis include arterial thrombosis (including myocardial infarction, stroke, leg ischaemia), lactic acidosis and cerebral oedema. Lactic acidosis is associated with ketoacidosis in patients with circulatory shock, severe sepsis, necrotising inflammation or when metformin is used.

72.   A. F   B. T   C. F   D. F   E. T

Sulphonylureas are indicated for non-pregnant adults with NIDDM and mild to moderate hyperglycaemia. It should not be used in children, during pregnancy or lactation. Insulin therapy should be used in pregnant patients when dietary modification is not adequate. Metformin may be useful in those with associated hyperlipidaemia, as the drug may promote a reduction of LDL-cholesterol and triglycerides while increasing HDL-cholesterol. Metformin is also useful in the treatment of obese patients with NIDDM. Sulphonylureas are preferred in patients with hyperglycaemic exacerbations, whilst metformin is useful in those prone to hypoglycaemia. Combined therapy with sulphonylurea and metformin may be used as an alternative to insulin. The mechanism of action of these drugs is separate and complementary and in combination may be effective in patients who do not achieve euglycaemia with either drug alone. Chlorpropamide like other sulphonylureas may cause disulfiram reaction in alcoholic patients.

73. *Fasting hypoglycaemia may be seen in*

A. insulinoma.
B. severe hepatic disease.
C. alcohol intoxication.
D. adrenal insufficiency.
E. Cushing's syndrome.

A........... B.......... C.......... D.......... E..........

74. *Recognised causes of hyperthyroidism include*

A. Graves' disease.
B. toxic multinodular goitre.
C. single thyroid adenoma.
D. subacute thyroiditis.
E. chronic β-blocker therapy.

A........... B.......... C.......... D.......... E..........

75. *Increase in thyroxine-binding globulin (TBG) levels are a feature of*

A. nephrotic syndrome.
B. androgen therapy.
C. pregnancy.
D. chronic active hepatitis.
E. oestrogen therapy.

A........... B.......... C.......... D.......... E..........

76. *The following statements about plasma TSH assay are correct.*

A. A normal TSH assay excludes both hyperthyroidism and primary hypothyroidism with a high degree of certainty.
B. TSH levels are useful in the diagnosis of secondary hypothyroidism.
C. Abnormal TSH levels are not specific for clinically important thyroid disease.
D. TSH levels may be suppressed in non-thyroidal illness.
E. Plasma TSH may be mildly elevated in some euthyroid patients with non-thyroidal illness and in subclinical hypothyroidism.

A........... B.......... C.......... D.......... E..........

77. *The following associations between non-thyroidal conditions and their effect on thyroid function tests are correct.*

A. Low T_3 syndrome–after trauma.
B. Low T_4 syndrome–severe illness.
C. High T_4 syndrome–psychiatric illness.
D. Hyperthyroidism–amiodarone.
E. Hypothyroidism–amiodarone.

A........... B.......... C.......... D.......... E..........

73.   A. T   B. T   C. T   D. T   E. F

Fasting hypoglycaemia is seen in insulinoma (β-cell tumours), severe hepatic disease, alcohol intoxication, adrenal insufficiency, hypothyroidism, growth hormone deficiency, hypofunction of pituitary, extrapancreatic neoplasms, partial gastrectomy and malnutrition.

74.   A. T   B. T   C. T   D. T   E. F

Causes of hyperthyroidism include Graves' disease, toxic multinodular goitre, single thyroid adenoma and subacute thyroiditis.

75.   A. F   B. F   C. T   D. T   E. T

Increase in TBG levels are is seen in pregnancy, oestrogen therapy, chronic active hepatitis and familial TBG excess. Low TBG levels are seen in severe liver disease, nephrotic syndrome, androgen therapy, severe malnutrition and familial TBG deficiency.

76.   A. T   B. F   C. T   D. T   E. T

Plasma TSH assay is the most useful diagnostic test in patients with suspected thyroidal disorders. Newer TSH assays are able to measure levels to a detection limit of $0.1\,\mu U\,ml^{-1}$. TSH levels are elevated in primary hypothyroidism and suppressed in hyperthyroidism. In suspected primary hypothyroidism, a normal TSH value excludes the condition and a markedly elevated level confirms the diagnosis. In secondary hypothyroidism (due to TSH deficiency) the TSH levels are usually within normal range and hence this assay is not useful for detection of this rare form of hypothyroidism. A normal TSH assay excludes both hyperthyroidism and primary hypothyroidism with a high degree of certainty. Abnormal TSH levels are not specific for clinically important thyroid disease because even small changes in thyroid hormone levels affect TSH secretion and hence the presence of thyroid disease should be confirmed by plasma serum thyroxine (T_4) and triiodothyronine (T_3) levels. TSH levels may be suppressed in non-thyroidal illness, by high-dose glucocorticoid therapy or dopamine treatment, in euthyroid elderly patients or in subclinical hyperthyroidism. Plasma TSH may be mildly elevated in some euthyroid patients with non-thyroidal illness and in subclinical hypothyroidism.

77.   A. T   B. T   C. T   D. T   E. T

The low T_3 syndrome occurs following trauma including surgery, during starvation and most illness. Plasma T_3 levels are low because the conversion of serum T_4 to T_3 is decreased. In severe illness, serum T_4 is low due to any of the following: suppression of TSH secretion, decrease in TBG levels and inhibition of T_4 binding to TBG. In psychiatric illness or acute medical emergencies, a high T_4 level may be seen and this is often due to increased TBG levels. Amiodarone and radiocontrast agents may cause either hyperthyroidism or hypothyroidism.

78. *The following statements about the management of hypothyroidism are correct.*

   A. In primary hypothyroidism, the goal of therapy is to maintain plasma TSH within the normal range.
   B. In secondary hypothyroidism, plasma TSH cannot be used to adjust therapy.
   C. Coronary artery disease may be exacerbated by the treatment of hypothyroidism.
   D. Thyroid hormone replacement in hypothyroidism may exacerbate any associated adrenal failure.
   E. Annual follow-up is required in patients undergoing treatment for hypothyroidism.

   A........... B.......... C.......... D.......... E..........

79. *The following statements about the management of hyperthyroidism are correct.*

   A. Propranolol is the definitive therapy in most adults with Graves' disease.
   B. Radioactive iodine therapy is the treatment of choice for most non-pregnant adults.
   C. In the majority of patients with Graves' disease, hyperthyroidism recurs after propylthiouracil is stopped.
   D. Amiodarone-induced hyperthyroidism is treated with subtotal thyroidectomy.
   E. Routine monitoring of white blood cell (WBC) count is useful in detecting agranulocytosis associated with antithyroid drugs.

   A........... B.......... C.......... D.......... E..........

80. *The following statements about euthyroid goitre are correct.*

   A. Most euthyroid goitres in the UK are due to Hashimoto's thyroiditis.
   B. Most multinodular goitres require no treatment.
   C. The risk of malignancy in multinodular goitres is very high.
   D. All single thyroid nodules should be evaluated with needle aspiration biopsy.
   E. Hoarseness due to vocal cord paralysis in patients with solitary nodule suggests malignancy.

   A........... B.......... C.......... D.......... E..........

78.   A. T   B. T   C. T   D. T   E. T

In primary hypothyroidism, the goal of therapy is to maintain plasma TSH within the normal range. As it takes months for TSH levels to return to normal, follow-up TSH levels should be measured 3–4 months following initiation of thyroxine therapy. In secondary hypothyroidism, plasma TSH cannot be used to adjust therapy and the goal of therapy is to maintain plasma T_4 index in the middle of the reference range. Coronary artery disease may be exacerbated by the treatment of hypothyroidism and treatment in such patients is started at low doses and increments are made slowly; care is taken to detect worsening of heart failure, angina or arrhythmias. Thyroid hormone replacement in hypothyroidism may exacerbate any associated adrenal failure. In such patients the development of orthostatic hypotension, nausea or vomiting after initiation of thyroxine therapy should prompt investigation for adrenal failure. Annual follow-up is required in patients undergoing treatment for hypothyroidism, with measurement of plasma TSH to allow adjustment of dose.

79.   A. F   B. T   C. T   D. F   E. F

Propranolol is used to control symptoms (tremor, palpitations and anxiety) in Graves' disease until definitive therapy takes effect. Radioactive iodine therapy is the treatment of choice for most non-pregnant adults. In the majority of patients with Graves' disease, hyperthyroidism recurs after propylthiouracil is stopped. Amiodarone-induced hyperthyroidism is treated with propylthiouracil and β-blockers. Although subtotal thyroidectomy provides long-term control of hyperthyroidism in most patients, because of the risk of surgical morbidity and mortality it is reserved only for those unwilling to undergo radioiodine therapy whose symptoms are not controlled by antithyroid drugs. Routine monitoring of WBC count is not useful in detecting agranulocytosis associated with antithyroid drugs. Agranulocytosis should be suspected when patients develop fever, sore throat, chills or bleeding gums.

80.   A. T   B. T   C. F   D. T   E. T

Most euthyroid goitres in the UK are due to Hashimoto's thyroiditis. Most multinodular goitres require no treatment. The risk of malignancy in multinodular goitres is very low when compared with the risk of thyroid carcinoma in clinically normal glands. However, patients with multinodular goitre should be evaluated for carcinoma if even one nodule enlarges disproportionately compared with the rest of the gland. All single thyroid nodules should be evaluated with needle aspiration biopsy. Hoarseness due to vocal cord paralysis in patients with solitary nodule suggests malignancy.

81. *Recognised causes of adrenal cortical failure include*

A. Autoimmune deficiency syndrome (AIDS).
B. phaeochromocytoma.
C. tuberculosis.
D. withdrawal of long-term glucocorticoid therapy.
E. Cushing's syndrome.

A.......... B.......... C.......... D.......... E..........

82. *Recognised features of patients with primary adrenal failure include*

A. ACTH levels are not detectable.
B. hyperpigmentation.
C. hyperkalaemia.
D. loss of visual fields.
E. orthostatic hypotension.

A.......... B.......... C.......... D.......... E..........

83. *Recognised features of Cushing's syndrome include*

A. amenorrhoea.
B. diabetes mellitus.
C. fat deposits in the supraclavicular fossae.
D. osteoporosis.
E. proximal muscle weakness.

A.......... B.......... C.......... D.......... E..........

84. *The following statements about the aetiology of Cushing's syndrome are correct.*

A. Hyperpigmentation excludes ectopic ACTH secretion.
B. Hypokalaemic alkalosis excludes ectopic ACTH secretion.
C. Glucocorticoid therapy is the most common cause of Cushing's syndrome.
D. ACTH-secreting pituitary microadenomas account for the majority of cases of endogenous Cushing's syndrome.
E. Hirsutism is not common in Cushing's syndrome caused by exogenous steroids.

A.......... B.......... C.......... D.......... E..........

85. *The following statements about the investigation of Cushing's syndrome are correct.*

A. A normal overnight dexamethasone test excludes the diagnosis.
B. Random plasma cortisol levels are useful in making the diagnosis.
C. A normal 24-h urinary cortisol test excludes the diagnosis.
D. Severe depression may cause false-positive dexamethasone suppression test.
E. Corticotrophin-releasing hormone test is helpful in distinguishing pituitary-led Cushing's disease from ectopic ACTH secretion.

A.......... B.......... C.......... D.......... E..........

81.   A. T   B. F   C. T   D. T   E. F

Autoimmune disorders, which may be associated with other endocrine conditions such as hypothyroidism and hypoparathyroidism, are the commonest cause of primary adrenal failure. Tuberculosis and histoplasmosis of the adrenal glands can cause adrenal failure. Patients with AIDS can develop adrenal failure due to fungal or mycobacterial infection, lymphoma of the adrenals or treatment with ketoconazole, which inhibits steroid synthesis. Glucocorticoid therapy may suppress ACTH for a year after steroid therapy is stopped, resulting in adrenal failure.

82.   A. F   B. T   C. T   D. F   E. T

In both primary and secondary adrenal failure there is hyponatraemia, orthostatic hypotension, anorexia, nausea, vomiting and weight loss. Hyperpigmentation and hyperkalaemia indicate primary adrenal involvement. Secondary adrenal failure causes deficiency of cortisol, but not aldosterone; hyperkalaemia and hyperpigmentation do not occur, although life-threatening adrenal crisis may develop. Visual field deficits are associated with pituitary tumours and are features of secondary adrenal failure.

83.   A. T   B. T   C. T   D. T   E. T

Clinical features of Cushing's syndrome include moon-like rounded face, hirsutism, deposits of fat over the posterior part of the neck and supraclavicular fossae, truncal obesity, amenorrhoea, depression, thin, easily bruisable skin, reddish striae, proximal muscle weakness, osteoporosis, impaired glucose tolerance and diabetes mellitus.

84.   A. F   B. F   C. T   D. T   E. T

Glucocorticoid therapy is the most common cause of Cushing's syndrome. Hirsutism is not common in Cushing's syndrome caused by exogenous steroids because they suppress adrenal androgen secretion. ACTH-secreting pituitary microadenomas account for 80% of the cases of endogenous Cushing's syndrome. Cushing's disease is increased production by the adrenals secondary to excess pituitary ACTH whereas Cushing's syndrome is caused by excess steroid from any cause. Ectopic ACTH secretion and adrenal tumours account only for a small proportion of cases.

85.   A. T   B. F   C. T   D. T   E. T

Random plasma urinary cortisol levels are not useful in making a diagnosis of Cushing's syndrome because the wide range of normal values overlaps those seen in this condition. Both 24-h urinary cortisol levels and overnight dexamethasone suppression test are very sensitive and a normal value excludes the diagnosis. In chronic alcoholic patients and patients with depression there may be increased urinary excretion of steroids, absent diurnal variation of plasma steroids and a positive overnight dexamethasone test. Corticotrophin-releasing hormone test is helpful in distinguishing pituitary-led Cushing's disease from ectopic ACTH secretion.

86. *Recognised causes of hyperpigmentation include*

A. uraemia.
B. primary biliary cirrhosis.
C. Nelson's syndrome.
D. haemochromatosis.
E. malabsorption syndrome.

A..........   B..........   C..........   D..........   E..........

87. *Recognised features of acromegaly include*

A. carpal tunnel syndrome.
B. increased mortality from cardiovascular disease.
C. bitemporal hemianopia.
D. acanthosis nigricans.
E. microglossia.

A..........   B..........   C..........   D..........   E..........

88. *The following statements about hyperprolactinaemia are correct.*

A. In women the most common pathological cause is pituitary macroadenoma.
B. In men the most common cause is prolactin-secreting pituitary microadenoma.
C. Hyperprolactinaemia in men causes gynaecomastia.
D. In women it causes amenorrhoea.
E. Prolactin is elevated in myxoedema.

A..........   B..........   C..........   D..........   E..........

89. *Hypercalcaemia*

A. is usually due to hyperparathyroidism in patients seen in an outpatient setting.
B. is usually due to malignancy in patients seen in hospitals.
C. can be caused by diuretics in patients with increased bone turnover.
D. in most patients is due to sarcoidosis.
E. increases the risk of digitalis toxicity.

A..........   B..........   C..........   D..........   E..........

90. *The following statements about the management of hypercalcaemia are correct.*

A. The first step is the replacement of extracellular volume with normal saline.
B. Pamidronate should be avoided.
C. Mithramycin should be used only in malignant hypercalcaemia.
D. Calcitonin should be avoided in renal failure.
E. Prednisone usually controls hypercalcaemia in multiple myeloma.

A..........   B..........   C..........   D..........   E..........

86.   A. T   B. T   C. T   D. T   E. T

Recognised causes of hyperpigmentation include Addison's disease, uraemia, primary biliary cirrhosis, Nelson's syndrome, haemochromatosis, malabsorption syndrome, sun-tan, race, porphyria cutanea tarda and ectopic ACTH syndrome.

87.   A. T   B. T   C. T   D. T   E. F

Acromegaly is almost always due to growth hormone excess secreted from a pituitary adenoma. Clinical features include enlargement of hands and feet, prominent supraorbital ridges, protrusion of the lower jaw, acanthosis nigricans and molluscum fibrosum in the axillae, hypertension, cardiomegaly, heart failure and increased mortality from cardiovascular disease. Bitemporal hemianopia is a feature of expanding pituitary tumour. Arthritis, carpal tunnel syndrome, spinal stenosis, hypertension, impaired glucose tolerance and macroglossia are other features of this condition.

88.   A. F   B. F   C. F   D. T   E. T

Pathological hyperprolactinaemia in women is either idiopathic or due to microadenomas, whereas in men it is due to macroadenomas. Other causes of hyperprolactinaemia include dopamine antagonists (phenothiazines, methyldopa, metoclopramide), verapamil, cimetidine, chronic renal failure and myxoedema. Hyperprolactinaemia causes amenorrhoea and infertility in women, and androgen deficiency and infertility but not gynaecomastia in men. Microadenomas are treated because of infertility or to prevent oestrogen deficiency and the risk of osteoporosis. The treatment of choice is the dopamine agonist bromocriptine, which suppresses plasma prolactin. In macroadenomas the patients are treated initially with bromocriptine to reduce both prolactin levels and tumour size, followed by trans-sphenoidal surgery if necessary.

89.   A. T   B. T   C. T   D. F   E. T

Hypercalcaemia is usually due to hyperparathyroidism in patients seen in an outpatient setting and due to malignancy in patients seen in hospitals. Drugs causing hypercalcaemia include diuretics, lithium and ingestion of large quantities of antacid. Uncommon causes include sarcoidosis, renal failure and prolonged immobilisation. Hypercalcaemia can shorten the QT interval and increase the risk of digitalis toxicity.

90.   A. T   B. F   C. T   D. F   E. T

Patients with hypercalcaemia are almost dehydrated and extracellular volume should be replaced with 0.9% saline. Pamidronate, an inhibitor of bone resorption, should be started early. Mithramycin should be used only in malignant hypercalcaemia. Calcitonin is rarely used but is administered in severe hypercalcaemia or renal failure. Prednisone usually controls hypercalcaemia in multiple myeloma and other haematological tumours. Parathyroidectomy is the only effective therapy in patients with primary hyperparathyroidism. Vitamin D intoxication should be treated with prednisone; hypercalcaemia of sarcoidosis also responds to prednisone.

91. *The following statements about osteoporosis are correct.*

    A. Postmenopausal osteoporosis is predominantly due to loss of cortical bone.
    B. In senile osteoporosis both cortical and trabecular bone are lost.
    C. Dual-energy radiography measures bone mass quantitatively.
    D. Oestrogen replacement is indicated for all women with premature menopause in the absence of contraindications.
    E. There is no well-established method of prevention or treatment of glucocorticoid-induced osteoporosis.

    A.......... B.......... C.......... D.......... E..........

92. *Recognised features of osteomalacia include the following.*

    A. It is associated with anticonvulsant therapy.
    B. Alkaline phosphatase levels are depressed.
    C. Both serum calcium and phosphorus are decreased.
    D. Looser's zones are seen on X-ray.
    E. Bone biopsy shows increased thickness of the osteoid seams.

    A.......... B.......... C.......... D.......... E..........

93. *Paget's disease of the bone*

    A. usually occurs before the age of 40.
    B. most often spares the pelvis, spine and skull.
    C. is a focal skeletal disorder.
    D. is associated with a depressed alkaline phosphatase level.
    E. is associated with high-output cardiac failure.

    A.......... B.......... C.......... D.......... E..........

94. *The following statements about the management of Paget's disease are correct.*

    A. Etidronate should be used if lytic disease of the weight-bearing bone is present.
    B. Most patients require no therapy.
    C. Calcitonin is indicated for treatment of fractures.
    D. Serum alkaline phosphatase levels should be measured during treatment.
    E. Human calcitonin is used if resistance to salmon calcitonin develops.

    A.......... B.......... C.......... D.......... E..........

91.   A. F   B. T   C. T   D. T   E. T

Postmenopausal osteoporosis (manifests usually 10 years after menopause) is predominantly due to loss of trabecular bone, resulting in Colles fractures of the distal forearm and fractures of vertebrae, loss of height, kyphosis and chronic back pain. In senile osteoporosis (manifests about the age of 70) both cortical and trabecular bone are lost, resulting in increased risk of fractures of the hip and vertebrae. Dual-energy radiography measures bone mass of the proximal femur and lumbar quantitatively with high precision and is used to determine the extent of osteopenia. Oestrogen replacement is indicated for all women with premature menopause in the absence of contraindications and should begin as soon as possible after menopause to delay the rapid phase of bone loss. However, the beneficial effects of oestrogen on bone mass, in those who attain menopause at the usual age, are evident until the age of 75. There is no well-established method of prevention or treatment of glucocorticoid-induced osteoporosis. Discontinuing steroid therapy if possible only partially reverses the glucocorticoid-induced bone loss.

92.   A. T   B. F   C. T   D. T   E. T

Osteomalacia due to vitamin D deficiency is associated with malabsorption, renal tubular acidosis, renal failure, therapy with anticonvulsants, fluoride, etidronate and hypophosphatasia. Both serum calcium and phosphorus levels are decreased, whereas alkaline phosphatase levels are elevated. Pseudofractures or Looser's zones are seen on radiographs of the chest, pelvis and hips. Serum 25-hydroxyvitamin D levels may be low. If neither these levels nor X-rays are diagnostic, bone biopsy may be required. Bone biopsy reveals increased thickness of the osteoid seams and decreased rate of mineralisation.

93.   A. F   B. F   C. T   D. F   E. T

Paget's disease of the bone usually occurs after the age of 40. It is a focal skeletal disorder associated with remodelling of bone and often affects the spine, pelvis, femur and skull. Most patients are discovered incidentally due to an elevated alkaline phosphatase level or when radiography is done for other indications. It may also manifest with deafness, arthritis, pathological fractures, high-output cardiac failure or osteogenic sarcoma.

94.   A. F   B. T   C. T   D. T   E. T

Most patients with Paget's disease require analgesia only or no therapy. Indications for therapy include specific complications such as bone pain, fractures, nerve compression, high-output cardiac failure, progressive bone deformity and immobilisation hypercalcaemia. Etidronate is usually the drug of choice and acts by inhibiting both bone resorption and formation. It should not be used if lytic disease of weight-bearing bones is present. Calcitonin is indicated for lytic disease of weight-bearing bone or when fractures are present. Human calcitonin is used if resistance to salmon calcitonin develops. Serum alkaline phosphatase levels are used to monitor therapy and a 50% reduction accompanied by an improvement of symptoms indicates an adequate response to treatment.

95.   *The following statements about hypocalcaemia are correct.*

   A. In hypoalbuminaemia with low serum total calcium, tetany occurs despite normal serum ionised calcium.
   B. Chronic hypocalcaemia may cause calcification of the basal ganglia.
   C. Serum parathormone is elevated in all causes of hypocalcaemia other than hypoparathyroidism and magnesium deficiency.
   D. Serum phosphorus levels are elevated in hypocalcaemia from most causes except vitamin D deficiency.
   E. Chvostek's sign excludes hypocalcaemia.

   A........... B.......... C.......... D.......... E..........

96.   *The following statements about glucose metabolism in pregnancy are correct.*

   A. Maternal insulin crosses the placenta.
   B. Pregnancy is an insulin-resistant state.
   C. Women with diabetic nephropathy should avoid pregnancy.
   D. Gestational diabetes causes excessive fetal insulin secretion.
   E. About two-thirds of patients with gestational diabetes develop diabetes mellitus within 5 years of pregnancy.

   A........... B.......... C.......... D.......... E..........

97.   *The following statements about thyroid disease in pregnancy are correct.*

   A. Thyrotoxicosis increases risk of fetal loss.
   B. Hyperthyroidism is often more easily controlled in pregnant women.
   C. Methimazole causes aplasia cutis of the fetus.
   D. Maternal T_4 concentration should be maintained in the lower range of normal.
   E. Propylthiouracil is contraindicated as it crosses the placenta.

   A........... B.......... C.......... D.......... E..........

95.   A. F   B. T   C. T   D. T   E. F

Hypoalbuminaemia is the most common cause of low total serum calcium but if the free (or ionised) level of calcium in the serum is normal there is no disorder of calcium metabolism. Tetany in hypocalcaemia may be latent and can be elicited by tapping anterior to the ear, which causes twitching of facial muscles (Chvostek's sign), or by inflating the blood pressure cuff above systolic pressure for 3 min, which causes spasm of the hand (Trousseau's sign). Chronic hypocalcaemia may be asymptomatic but may cause cataracts or calcification of the basal ganglia. Serum parathormone is elevated in all causes of hypocalcaemia other than hypoparathyroidism and magnesium deficiency. Serum phosphorus levels are elevated in hypocalcaemia from most causes except vitamin D deficiency.

96.   A. F   B. T   C. F   D. T   E. F

Pregnancy resembles starvation in that ketoacidosis develops in the absence of striking hyperglycaemia seen in diabetic patients. Maternal glucagon and insulin do not cross the placenta, but acetoacetate and β-hydroxybutyrate cross readily and are oxidised by the fetal liver and brain. Despite the fetal demand for glucose, pregnancy is a diabetogenic state due to insulin resistance (due to elevation of hormones such as oestrogen, progesterone, prolactin and human placental lactogen). Pregnancy in diabetic patients is associated with a higher perinatal mortality and a higher incidence of congenital anomalies. Gestational diabetes results in increased fetal insulin secretion, which in turn can cause macrosomia and increased risk for birth trauma and the need for a Caesarean. Patients with diabetic nephropathy usually have a normal pregnancy, although the patients require more care. Usually glucose tolerance returns to normal following delivery in patients with gestational diabetes but one-third or more develop frank diabetes mellitus within 5 years of pregnancy.

97.   A. F   B. T   C. T   D. F   E. F

Thyrotoxicosis does not increase fetal loss nor does pregnancy worsen thyrotoxicosis; in fact, hyperthyroidism is often more easily controlled during pregnancy. Methimazole should be avoided as it can cause aplasia cutis of the fetus. Propylthiouracil is the drug of choice but the dose should be kept as low as possible (with maternal T_4 levels being maintained in the upper range of normal) as it crosses the placenta causing fetal goitre.

98. *The following statements about defective transmembrane signalling are correct.*

 A. Laron dwarfism is due to growth hormone receptor defects.
 B. Familial hypercholesterolaemia is due to defective HDL-cholesterol gene.
 C. Leprechaunism is due to loss of signal transduction through the insulin receptor.
 D. NIDDM exhibits a defect in GLUT4 receptors.
 E. Achondroplasia is due to defects in the fibroblast growth factor receptor gene.

 A.......... B.......... C.......... D.......... E..........

99. *The following statements are correct.*

 A. Tyrosinaemia is due to fumarylacetoacetate hydrolase defect.
 B. Homocystinuria is due to cystathione B synthase deficiency.
 C. Lesch–Nyhan syndrome is due to hypoxanthine phosphoribosyltransferase deficiency.
 D. Adult Refsum's disease is due to phytanic acid α-hydroxylase deficiency.
 E. Lactic acidosis can be due to a defect in pyruvate dehydrogenase.

 A.......... B.......... C.......... D.......... E..........

100. *The following associations are correct*

 A. C1 esterase inhibitor–angioneurotic oedema.
 B. α_1-antitrypsin–pulmonary emphysema and or cirrhosis.
 C. Caeruloplasmin–Wilson's disease.
 D. Somatomedin–pituitary dwarfism.
 E. Mevolanate kinase–isovaleric acidaemia.

 A.......... B.......... C.......... D.......... E..........

101. *Insulin promotes glucose storage*

 A. brain.
 B. red blood cells.
 C. myocardium.
 D. skeletal muscle.
 E. liver.

 A.......... B.......... C.......... D.......... E..........

98.   A. T   B. F   C. T   D. T   E. T

Laron dwarfism results from growth hormone receptor defects and its
manifestations include proportionate dwarfism, hypoglycaemia, frontal bossing,
balding, truncal obesity and wrinkled skin. Familial hypercholesterolaemia is
associated with decreased number or function of the LDL receptors and the loss
of the cell's ability to down-regulate endogenous cholesterol synthesis. This
results in increased intracellular and intravascular accumulation of LDL-
cholesterol with resultant atherosclerosis and heart disease. Leprechaunism is a
rare disorder of severe insulin resistance where affected infants have low birth
weight, acanthosis nigricans, cystic changes in organs and loss of glucose
homeostasis. More than one glucose transporter is expressed by most cells. For
example, jejunal epithelial cells accumulate glucose at the luminal surface using
SGLT-1 and expel glucose at the basolateral surface through the glucose
transporter GLUT-2. An insulin-responsive, facilitative glucose transporter
(GLUT-4) is not sodium-dependent and is expressed primarily in insulin-
responsive tissues (fat cells, skeletal muscle); along with GLUT-2 it is defective in
NIDDM. Achondroplasia is an autosomal co-dominant trait with complete
penetrance. Mutations of the fibroblast growth factor receptor 3 (FGFR-3) gene
with the transition from guanine to adenine or a guaninie to cytosine
transversion at nucleotide 1138 is the defect in these patients

99.   A. T   B. T   C. T   D. T   E. T

Tyrosinaemia is either due to a deficiency of fumarylacetoacetate hydrolase or
that of tyrosine aminotransferase. When due to fumarylacetoacetate hydrolase
deficiency it is an autosomal recessive condition and manifests with
succinylaccetone accumulation with acute porphyria. Homocystinuria is an
autosomal recessive condition and is due to cystathione B synthase deficiency. It
manifests with marfanoid habitus, arterial thrombosis, lens dislocation and
mental retardation. Lesch–Nyhan syndrome has an X-linked inheritance and is
due to hypoxanthine phosphoribosyltransferase deficiency and manifestations
include neurologic dysfunction with self-destructive tendency. Lactic acidosis
can be due to a defect in pyruvate hydrogenase or in pyruvate decarboxylase.
Adult Refsum's disease is due to phytanic acid deficiency.

100.   A. T   B. T   C. T   D. T   E. F

Isovaleric acidemia is due to a defect in isovaleryl CoA dehydrogenase.
Angioneurotic oedema is due to a deficiency in C1 esterase inhibitor, alpha-1
antitrypsin deficiency results in pulmonary emphysema and cirrhosis. Wilson's
disease is associated with low serum ceruloplasmin and Laron dwarfism is due to
somatomedin deficiency.

101.   A. F   B. F   C. T   D. T   E. T

Insulin regulates glucose storage in most tissues except brain and red blood cells.

102. *Glucagon*

A. is secreted by the islet β cells of the pancreas.
B. is used in the treatment of hypoglycaemia.
C. promotes glycogen storage by the liver.
D. is used in overdose due to β-adrenergic blockers.
E. is used in overdose due to calcium channel blockers.

A............   B..........   C..........   D..........   E..........

103. *TSH stimulates thyroid function by increasing*

A. rate of synthesis of thyroglobulin.
B. synthesis of TBG.
C. iodine uptake by the thyroid from the blood.
D. iodination of tyrosine.
E. size of the thyroid gland.

A............   B..........   C..........   D..........   E..........

104. *The following hormones enter the cell to mediate their effects.*

A. cortisol.
B. insulin.
C. growth hormone.
D. glucagon.
E. parathyroid hormone.

A............   B..........   C..........   D..........   E..........

105. *Oestrogens cause*

A. growth of hair in the pubic region.
B. milk secretion by the alveoli of the breasts.
C. deposition of fat in the breasts.
D. enlargement of external genitalia.
E. skin to develop a soft texture.

A............   B..........   C..........   D..........   E..........

106. *Ejection of milk from the breast*

A. can occur from both breasts although the baby is nursing only one breast.
B. is regulated by aldosterone.
C. can occur by mechanical stimulation of the nipple.
D. can be stimulated by the sight of the baby.
E. is regulated by oxytocin.

A............   B..........   C..........   D..........   E..........

102.   A. F   B. T   C. F   D. T   E. T

Glucagon is secreted by the α cells of the islets of Langerhans of the pancreas. It is used in the management of hypoglycaemia and in overdose due to β-blockers and calcium channel blockers. It promotes glycogenolysis in the liver.

103.   A. T   B. F   C. T   D. T   E. T

TSH has no effect on TBG, which is not produced in the thyroid gland. All the other reactions occur in the thyroid and are enhanced by TSH.

104.   A. T   B. F   C. F   D. F   E. F

All the hormones except cortisol mediate their effects by stimulating receptors on the cell membrane and activating a second messenger system, whereas steroids such as cortisol must enter the nucleus to cause their effects.

105.   A. F   B. F   C. T   D. T   E. T

Growth of pubic hair is caused by androgens. Oestrogens do not promote milk secretion by the alveoli but do promote deposition of fat in the breasts, enlargement of external genitalia and the skin to develop a soft texture.

106.   A. T   B. F   C. T   D. T   E. T

'Let down' or ejection of milk from the breast can occur from both breasts although the baby is nursing only one breast. It can occur by the sight or sound of the baby and by mechanical stimulation of the nipple. It is regulated by oxytocin.

3 GENETIC DISORDERS AND IMMUNOLOGY

107. *The following statements are correct.*

    A. Phenylketonuria is due to a splice site mutation.
    B. Tay–Sachs disease is due to a frameshift mutation.
    C. Cystic fibrosis is due to a three-base deletion.
    D. Hereditary haemolytic anaemia is due to mutations within noncoding sequences.
    E. Sickle cell haemoglobin is due to a point mutation.

    A.......... B.......... C.......... D.......... E..........

108. *The following statements about most autosomal recessive disorders are correct.*

    A. Complete penetrance is rare.
    B. Onset is frequently late in life.
    C. New mutations are rarely detected clinically.
    D. The trait does not usually affect the parents, but siblings may show the disease.
    E. The proband is almost never a product of consanguineous marriage.

    A.......... B.......... C.......... D.......... E..........

109. *Familial hypercholesterolaemia*

    A. is the most frequent Mendelian disorder.
    B. is the consequence of a mutation in the gene encoding the receptor for HDL.
    C. is associated with premature atherosclerosis.
    D. is associated with a greatly increased risk of myocardial infarction.
    E. is associated with tendinous xanthomas.

    A.......... B.......... C.......... D.......... E..........

107.   A. T   B. T   C. T   D. T   E. T

When a single nucleotide base is substituted by a different base, resulting in partial or complete deletion of a gene, it is known as a point mutation, as in sickle cell anaemia. Here the nucleotide triplet CTC, which codes for glutamic acid, is changed to CAC, which codes for valine. This single amino acid substitution alters the physicochemical properties of haemoglobin, giving rise to sickle cell anaemia. Phenylketonuria is due to a splice site mutation of the gene for phenylalanine hydroxylase resulting in reduced amount of the enzyme. Small deletions or insertions involving the coding sequence lead to alterations in the reading frame of the DNA strand, referred to as frameshift mutations. A four-base insertion in the hexosaminidase A gene in Tay–Sachs disease leads to a frameshift mutation. This mutation is the major cause of Tay–Sachs disease in Ashkenazi Jews. Three-base deletion in the common cystic fibrosis allele results in synthesis of a protein that is missing amino acid 508 (phenylalanine). Because the deletion is a multiple of three, this is not a frameshift mutation. Mutations within non-coding sequences, such as the promoter or enhancer sequences, lead to marked reduction in, or total lack of, transcription as in certain forms of hereditary haemolytic anaemias. Huntington's disease is not due to a point mutation.

108.   A. F   B. F   C. T   D. T   E. F

Autosomal recessive disorders result only when both alleles at a given locus are mutants. Such disorders are characterised by the following features: (1) the trait does not usually affect the parents, but siblings may show the disease; (2) siblings have a one in four chance of being affected; and (3) the mutant gene occurs with a low frequency in the population and thus, there is a strong likelihood that the proband is the product of a consanguineous marriage. Complete penetrance is more common and the onset is frequently early in life. Although new mutations for recessive disorders do occur they are rarely detected clinically.

109.   A. T   B. F   C. T   D. T   E. T

Familial hypercholesterolaemia is the consequence of a mutation in the gene encoding the receptor for LDL, which is involved in the transport and metabolism of cholesterol. It is possibly the most frequent Mendelian disorder. Heterozygotes, with one mutant gene, represent about 1 in 500 individuals. From birth they have a two- to three-fold elevation of plasma cholesterol, leading to tendinous xanthomas, premature atherosclerosis in adult life and a greatly increased risk of myocardial infarction. Homozygotes are more severely affected and have a five- to six-fold elevation of plasma cholesterol levels. These individuals develop cutaneous xanthomas and coronary, cerebral and peripheral vascular atherosclerosis at an early age. Myocardial infarction may develop before the age of 20 years.

110. *Recognised features of Marfan's syndrome include the following:*

A. it results from mutations of the fibrillin gene.
B. ectopia lentis.
C. aortic stenosis.
D. autosomal recessive inheritance.
E. presymptomatic detection is possible by restriction fragment length polymorphism analysis.

A............   B..........   C..........   D..........   E..........

111. *Recognised features of Ehlers–Danlos syndromes include the following:*

A. the skin is hyperextensible.
B. the joints are hypermobile.
C. it results from a defect in elastin.
D. the mode of inheritance encompasses all three Mendelian patterns.
E. hypercholesterolaemia.

A............   B..........   C..........   D..........   E..........

112. *Tay–Sachs disease*

A. is due to accumulation of sphingomyelin.
B. is due to a deficiency of hexosaminidase A.
C. is prevalent in Ashkenazi Jews.
D. is characterised by a cherry-red spot in the macula.
E. patients have a normal life span.

A............   B..........   C..........   D..........   E..........

110. A. T   B. T   C. F   D. F   E. T

Marfan's syndrome is a disorder of the connective tissues of the body, manifested by changes in the skeleton, eyes and cardiovascular system. It is the result of mutations in the fibrillin gene. Fibrillin is a glycoprotein secreted by fibroblasts that aggregates either alone or in conjunction with other proteins to form a microfibrillar network in the extracellular matrix. Recognised features include unusually long, slender extremities and tall stature contributed largely by the lower segment of the body. Bilateral subluxation or dislocation of the lens, referred to as ectopia lentis, is characteristic of this condition. Loss of medial support results in progressive dilatation of the aortic valve ring and the root of the aorta, giving rise to severe aortic regurgitation. Presymptomatic detection is possible by restriction fragment length polymorphism analysis.

111. A. T   B. T   C. F   D. T   E. F

Ehlers–Danlos syndromes comprise a clinically and genetically heterogeneous group of disorders that result from some defect in collagen synthesis or structure. There are at least 10 different variants of this syndrome due to the fact there are at least 12 genetically different collagen types, each with somewhat characteristic tissue distribution. The mode of inheritance of this syndrome encompasses all three Mendelian patterns. Because the abnormal collagen fibres lack adequate tensile strength, skin is hyperextensible and the joints are hypermobile. These disorders are extremely heterogeneous, although the common thread is some abnormality in collagen. At the molecular level, a variety of defects, varying from mutations involving structural genes for collagen to those involving enzymes that are responsible for post-transcriptional modifications of mRNA, have been detected.

112. A. F   B. T   C. T   D. T   E. F

Tay–Sachs disease is due to mutations that affect the α-subunit locus on chromosome 15, which cause a severe deficiency of hexosaminidase A. This enzyme is absent from virtually all tissues including leucocytes and plasma; thus GM2 ganglioside accumulates in many tissues (including heart, liver and spleen), but the involvement of neurones in the central and autonomic nervous systems and retina dominates the picture. A cherry-red spot appears in the macula, representing accentuation of the normal colour of the macular choroid contrasted with pallor produced by the swollen ganglion cells. Although not pathognomonic, it is seen in almost all patients. This disease is particularly prevalent in Ashkenazi Jews and typically has relentless motor and mental deterioration followed by death at the age of 2 or 3 years.

113. *In Niemann–Pick disease*

    A. there is lysosomal accumulation of sphingomyelin.
    B. clinical manifestations may present even at birth.
    C. the liver and spleen shrink.
    D. there is increased activity of the enzyme sphingomyelinase in the liver.
    E. carriers can be detected by DNA probe analysis.

    A............ B........... C........... D........... E...........

114. *Gaucher's disease is*

    A. an autosomal dominant disorder.
    B. rare in Jews.
    C. characterised by increased glucocerebrosidase activity.
    D. characterised by massive splenomegaly.
    E. diagnosed by measurement of glucocerebrosidase activity in peripheral blood leucocytes.

    A............ B........... C........... D........... E...........

115. *The following associations regarding glycogen storage diseases are correct.*

    A. McArdle's syndrome–painful muscle cramps.
    B. von Gierke's disease–hepatomegaly.
    C. Pompe's disease–massive cardiomegaly.
    D. Pompe's disease–deficiency of acid maltase.
    E. von Gierke's disease–deficiency of glucose 6-phosphatase.

    A............ B........... C........... D........... E...........

116. *Skeletal abnormalities seen in neurofibromatosis include*

    A. scoliosis.
    B. subperiosteal bone cysts.
    C. pseudoarthrosis of the tibia.
    D. intraosseous cystic lesions.
    E. Looser's zones.

    A............ B........... C........... D........... E...........

117. *Patients with neurofibromatosis have two- to four-fold greater risk of developing*

    A. mesothelioma.
    B. bronchogenic carcinoma.
    C. meningiomas.
    D. optic gliomas.
    E. phaeochromocytomas.

    A............ B........... C........... D........... E...........

113. A. T   B. T   C. F   D. F   E. T

Niemann–Pick disease refers to a group of disorders that are clinically, biochemically and genetically heterogeneous but all have lysosomal accumulation of sphingomyelin and cholesterol. There is deficiency of sphingomyelinase and the diagnosis is established by biochemical assays for sphingomyelinase activity in liver or bone marrow biopsy. The sphingomyelinase gene has been cloned and hence individuals affected as well as carriers can be detected by DNA probe analysis. Clinical features may be present even at birth and are certainly evident by 6 months of age. Manifestations include hepatosplenomegaly, skin xanthomas, lymphadenopathy and progressive failure to thrive with deterioration of psychomotor function. Death usually occurs within the second year of life.

114. A. F   B. F   C. F   D. T   E. T

Gaucher's disease is an autosomal recessive disorder resulting from mutations at the glucocerebrosidase locus on chromosome 1. There is deficiency of glucocerebrosidase, an enzyme that normally cleaves the glucose residue from ceramide. This results in the accumulation of glucocerebroside in the phagocytic cells of the body and in the CNS. Massive splenomegaly and hypersplenism are important features of this disease. Other manifestations include pathological fractures and CNS dysfunction. The diagnosis in homozygotes can be made by measurement of glucocerebrosidase activity in peripheral blood leucocytes. However, there is considerable overlap between enzyme levels in normal and heterozygote patients, where detection of specific mutations is required.

115. A. T   B. T   C. T   D. T   E. T

von Gierke's disease is the hepatic type of glycogen storage disease and is due to deficiency of glucose 6-phosphatase. Failure to thrive, hypoglycaemia, convulsions, gout, skin xanthomas, stunted growth, hepatomegaly and enlargement of the kidneys are important features. McArdle's syndrome or the myopathic type is due to a deficiency of muscle phosphorylase and is characterised by painful cramps associated with strenuous exercise and myoglobinuria; lifespan is normal. In Pompe's disease there is deficiency of acid maltase (lysosomal glucosidase) with mild hepatomegaly, cardiomegaly and skeletal muscle involvement.

116. A. T   B. T   C. T   D. T   E. T

About one-third to half the patients with neurofibromatosis have skeletal abnormalities, which include erosive defects due to contiguity of neurofibromas to the bone, scoliosis, intraosseous cystic lesions, subperiosteal bone cysts and pseudoarthrosis of the tibia.

117. A. F   B. F   C. T   D. T   E. T

Patients with neurofibromatosis have two- to four-fold greater risk of developing meningiomas, gliomas and phaeochromocytomas.

118. *The following statements about Down's syndrome are correct.*

A. The most common cause is meiotic non-disjunction.
B. The parents of children with trisomy 21 have a normal karyotype.
C. Maternal age has a strong influence on the incidence of Down's syndrome.
D. Most patients are mosaics.
E. Robertsonian translocation of the long arm of chromosome 21 to another acrocentric chromosome, e.g. 22 or 14, is a recognised mechanism.

A............   B...........   C...........   D...........   E...........

119. *The following statements about Down's syndrome are correct.*

A. Most have congenital heart disease.
B. Children with trisomy 21 have a 10–20-fold increased risk of developing acute leukaemia.
C. Virtually all patients with trisomy 21 older than the age of 40 develop dementia.
D. Patients have abnormal immune responses making them resistant to infections.
E. Currently more than four-fifths survive beyond the age of 30.

A............   B...........   C...........   D...........   E...........

120. *Recognised features of Down's syndrome include*

A. simian crease
B. abundant neck skin.
C. intestinal stenosis.
D. mental retardation.
E. hypotonia.

A............   B...........   C...........   D...........   E...........

121. *The Lyon hypothesis proposes that*

A. only one of the X chromosomes is genetically active.
B. the other X chromosome, either of maternal or paternal origin, undergoes pyknosis.
C. inactivation of either maternal or paternal X chromosome occurs at random among all cells of the blastocyst on or about the 16th day of embryonic life.
D. inactivation of the same X chromosome persists in all the cells derived from each precursor cell.
E. in general the higher the number of Y chromosomes, the greater the likelihood of mental retardation.

A............   B...........   C...........   D...........   E...........

118. A. T   B. T   C. T   D. F   E. T

The most common cause of Down's syndrome is trisomy 21 due to meiotic non-disjunction. The parents of such children have a normal karyotype and are normal in all respects. Maternal age has a strong influence on the incidence of Down's syndrome. It occurs in 1 in 1550 live births in women under the age of 20 years, in contrast to 1 in 25 live births for mothers over the age of 45. In 4% of all cases of Down's syndrome, extrachromosomal material derives from the presence of a Robertsonian translocation of the long arm of chromosome 21 to another acrocentric chromosome, e.g. 22 or 14. Such cases are frequently familial and the translocated chromosome is inherited from one of the parents who is a carrier of a Robertsonian translocation. Approximately 1% of Down's syndrome patients are mosaics, usually having a mixture of cells with 46 and 47 chromosomes. This results from mitotic non-disjunction of chromosome 21 during an early stage of embryogenesis.

119. A. F   B. T   C. T   D. F   E. T

Approximately two-fifths of patients with Down's syndrome have congenital heart disease, most commonly endocardial cushion defects including the ostium primum, atrial septal defect, atrioventricular malformations and ventricular septal defects. These are responsible for most of the deaths in infancy and early childhood. Children with trisomy 21 have a 10–20-fold increased risk of developing acute leukaemia. Virtually all patients with trisomy 21 older than the age of 40 develop dementia and the neuropathological changes are characteristic of Alzheimer's disease. Patients have abnormal immune responses making them susceptible to infections, particularly of the respiratory system, and to thyroid immunity. Currently more than four-fifths survive beyond the age of 30.

120. A. T   B. T   C. T   D. T   E. T

Down's syndrome is the leading cause of mental retardation and the presence of flat facial profile, oblique palpebral fissures and epicanthic folds accounts for the old designation of mongolian idiocy. It should be pointed out that some mosaics with Down's syndrome have very mild phenotypic changes and may even have normal or near-normal intelligence. Other features include simian crease, abundant neck skin, intestinal stenosis, hypotonia, gap between the first and second toe and umbilical hernia.

121. A. T   B. T   C. T   D. T   E. F

The Lyon hypothesis, outlined by British geneticist Mary Lyon, describes the inactivation of the X chromosome. It proposes that (1) only one of the X chromosomes is genetically active; (2) the other X chromosome either of maternal or paternal origin undergoes pyknosis; (3) inactivation of either maternal or paternal X chromosome occurs at random among all cells of the blastocyst on or about the 16th day of embryonic life; and (4) inactivation of the same X chromosome persists in all the cells derived from each precursor cell. Although the basic tenets of this hypothesis have stood the test of time, several modifications have been made including the fact that both X chromosomes are required for normal oogenesis.

122. *Klinefelter's syndrome*

A. occurs when supernumerary Y chromosomes are found in the male.
B. is the most common genetic cause of hypogonadism in the male.
C. is characterised by consistently elevated plasma gonadotrophin levels.
D. patients almost always have mental retardation.
E. is diagnosed rarely before puberty.

A........... B.......... C.......... D.......... E..........

123. *Recognised manifestations of Turner's syndrome include*

A. hypogonadism in a phenotypic female.
B. complete or partial monosomy of X chromosome.
C. coarctation of the aorta.
D. cubitus valgus.
E. low posterior hairline.

A........... B.......... C.......... D.......... E..........

124. *The following statements regarding hermaphroditism are correct.*

A. In true hermaphroditism both ovarian and testicular tissue are present.
B. Female pseudohermaphroditism is a feature of congenital adrenal hyperplasia.
C. Female pseudohermaphroditism is associated with normal ovaries.
D. Female pseudohermaphroditism is associated with virilized external genitalia.
E. Mutations of the androgen receptor result in male pseudohermaphroditism.

A........... B.......... C.......... D.......... E..........

125. *The following statements about mutations in mitochondrial genes are correct.*

A. The inheritance is paternal.
B. The deleterious effects are primarily on organs most dependent on oxidative phosphorylation.
C. Expression of disorders is quite variable.
D. Leber's hereditary optic atrophy is associated with mitochondrial inheritance.
E. Mendelian inheritance applies to these genes.

A........... B.......... C.......... D.......... E..........

122.   A. F   B. T   C. T   D. F   E. T

Klinefelter's syndrome is defined as male hypogonadism that occurs when there are two or more X chromosomes and one or more Y chromosomes. It is one of the most common causes of hypogonadism in the male. It can be diagnosed rarely before puberty, because the testicular abnormality does not develop before early puberty. Plasma gonadotrophin levels, particularly FSH, are consistently elevated and testosterone levels are variably reduced. There is considerable feminization and the mean intelligence quotient (IQ) is lower than normal, but mental retardation is uncommon.

123.   A. T   B. T   C. T   D. T   E. T

Turner's syndrome results from complete or partial monosomy of the X chromosome and is characterised primarily by hypogonadism in phenotypic females. Clinical features include short stature, broad chest and widely spaced nipples, webbing of the neck, cubitus valgus, peripheral lymph oedema at birth, coarctation of the aorta, streak ovaries, infertility, amenorrhoea and a low posterior hairline.

124.   A. T   B. T   C. T   D. T   E. T

In true hermaphroditism both ovarian and testicular tissue are present. Female pseudohermaphroditism is a feature of congenital adrenal hyperplasia and is associated with a genetic sex of XX and normal ovaries but with virilized external genitalia due to excess androgen secretion. In male pseudohermaphroditism the individuals possess a Y chromosome and thus their gonads are exclusively testis but the genital ducts or external genitalia are incompletely differentiated along the male phenotype. Mutations of the androgen receptor result in male pseudohermaphroditism.

125.   A. F   B. T   C. T   D. T   E. T

Mendelian inheritance applies to mitochondrial genes but the inheritance is maternal. The ovum contains abundant mitochondria unlike the spermatozoon and thus the mitochondrial complement of the zygote is almost entirely from the ovum. Mothers transmit mitochondrial DNA to all their offspring; however, daughters not sons transmit the DNA to further progeny. The deleterious effects are primarily on organs most dependent on oxidative phosphorylation, including skeletal muscle, CNS, cardiac muscle, liver and kidneys. As the mitochondria are randomly distributed during cell division, the expression of disorders due to mutations in mitochondrial DNA is quite variable. Leber's hereditary optic atrophy is associated with a mitochondrial inheritance and manifests with progressive bilateral loss of central vision, cardiac conduction defects and minor neurological defects.

126. *Complement-dependent reactions include*

    A. transfusions reactions in which cells from an incompatible donor react with autochthonous antibody of the host.

    B. erythroblastosis fetalis

    C. autoimmune haemolytic anaemia.

    D. atopy.

    E. Graves' disease.

    A.......... B.......... C.......... D.......... E..........

127. *The following statements about hypersensitivity reactions are correct.*

    A. In type I disease, the immune response releases vasoactive spasmogenic substances that act on vessels and smooth muscles.

    B. In type II disease, humoral antibodies participate directly in injuring cells by predisposing them to phagocytosis or lysis.

    C. In type III disorders or immune complex diseases, humoral antibodies bind antigens and activate complement, which in turn attract neutrophils that release enzymes causing tissue damage.

    D. In type IV disorders, cell-mediated immune responses with sensitised lymphocytes are the cause of cellular and tissue injury.

    E. Type I hypersensitivity reaction involves the combination of an antigen with antibody bound to mast cells in individuals previously sensitised to the antigen.

    A.......... B.......... C.......... D.......... E..........

128. *The following statements about histocompatibility antigens are correct.*

    A. The main function of the cell-surface molecules is to bind peptide fragments of foreign proteins for presentation to appropriate antigen-specific T cells.

    B. Class I antigens are expressed on all nucleated cells and platelets.

    C. Class II antigens are coded for in a region called HLA-D.

    D. Individuals who possess HLA-B27 antigen have a 90-fold greater chance of developing ankylosing spondylitis than those who are negative.

    E. Class II HLA antigens can regulate immune responsiveness.

    A.......... B.......... C.......... D.......... E..........

126. A. T   B. T   C. T   D. F   E. F

There are two mechanisms by which antibody and complement may mediate type II hypersensitivity: direct lysis and opsonisation. Clinically, such reactions occur in transfusion reactions, erythroblastosis fetalis, autoimmune haemolytic anaemia and certain drug reactions.

127. A. T   B. T   C. T   D. T   E. T

In type I disease, the immune response releases vasoactive spasmogenic substances that act on vessels and smooth muscles; in humans type I reactions are mediated by IgE antibodies. Type I hypersensitivity reaction involves the combination of an antigen with antibody bound to mast cells in individuals previously sensitised to the antigen. In type II disease, humoral antibodies participate directly in injuring cells by predisposing them to phagocytosis or lysis; type II hypersensitivity reactions are mediated by antibodies directed towards antigens present on the surface of cells or tissue components. In type III disorders or immune complex diseases, humoral antibodies bind antigens and activate complement, which in turn attract neutrophils that release enzymes causing tissue damage. In type IV disorders, cell-mediated immune responses with sensitised lymphocytes are the cause of cellular and tissue injury.

128. A. T   B. T   C. T   D. T   E. T

The main function of the cell-surface molecules is to bind peptide fragments of foreign proteins for presentation to appropriate antigen-specific T cells. Class I antigens are expressed on all nucleated cells and platelets. Class I antigens are encoded by three closely linked loci, designated HLA-A, HLA-B and HLA-C. Individuals who possess HLA-B27 antigen have a 90-fold greater chance of developing ankylosing spondylitis than those who are negative. Class II antigens are coded for in a region called HLA-D. Class II HLA antigens can regulate immune responsiveness.

129. *The following statements about graft survival are correct.*

A. In the case of kidney transplants from a related donor, a markedly beneficial effect of matching for class I antigens has been observed.

B. In cadaver renal transplants, matching for HLA class I antigens has at best a modest effect on graft acceptance.

C. Immunosuppressive therapy is unnecessary in graft recipients in HLA-identical siblings with minor histocompatibility loci.

D. Graft-versus-host disease occurs in any situation in which immunologically competent cells are transplanted into immunologically crippled recipients.

E. Depletion of donor T cells during bone marrow transplantation virtually eliminates graft-versus-host disease.

A...........   B..........   C..........   D..........   E..........

130. *The following associations in amyloidosis are correct.*

A. Long-term haemodialysis patients–deposition of β_2-microglobulin.

B. Multiple myeloma–AL amyloid.

C. Recurrent and chronic inflammation–AA amyloid.

D. Senile cardiac amyloidosis–ATTR amyloid.

E. Isolated atrial amyloidosis–AANF amyloid.

A...........   B..........   C..........   D..........   E..........

131. *The following statements about nuclear fluorescence are correct.*

A. Homogeneous or diffuse nuclear staining usually reflects antibodies to chromatin.

B. Rim or peripheral staining patterns are most commonly indicative of antibodies to double-stranded DNA.

C. Speckled patterns reflect the presence of antibodies to non-DNA nuclear constituents.

D. Nucleolar pattern is most reported in systemic sclerosis.

E. Speckled pattern is associated with extractable nuclear antigens.

A...........   B..........   C..........   D..........   E..........

129.   A. T   B. T   C. F   D. T   E. T

In the case of kidney transplants from a related donor, a markedly beneficial effect of matching for class I antigens has been observed. In cadaver renal transplants, matching for HLA class I antigens has at best a modest effect on graft acceptance. Immunosuppressive therapy is necessary in graft recipients even in HLA-identical siblings because several minor histocompatibility loci can evoke slow rejection. Graft-versus-host disease occurs in any situation in which immunologically competent cells are transplanted into immunologically crippled recipients. Because graft-versus-host disease is mediated by T lymphocytes contained in the donor bone marrow, depletion of donor T cells before transfusion, virtually eliminates graft-versus-host disease.

130.   A. T   B. T   C. T   D. T   E. T

Based on its constituent chemical fibrils amyloid is classified into categories such as AL, AA and ATTR. In multiple myeloma and other monoclonal B-cell proliferation, the major fibril protein is AL. The AL protein is composed of complete immunoglobulin light chains, the NH_2 fragments of light chains, or both. In recurrent and chronic inflammation and familial Mediterranean fever, the major fibril protein is AA. This second major class of amyloid fibril protein does not have structural homology to immunoglobulins but is derived from a larger precursor in the serum called serum amyloid-associated (SAA) protein that is synthesised in the liver and circulates in association with the HDL3 subclass of lipoproteins. In senile cardiac amyloidosis, the protein is ATTR and the chemically related precursor protein is transthyretin (also known as prealbumin). Transthyretin is a normal serum protein that binds and transports thyroxine and retinol. In isolated atrial amyloidosis, the major fibrillar protein is AANF and the chemically related precursor protein is atrial natriuretic factor. Patients on long-term haemodialysis for renal failure develop amyloidosis owing to deposition of β_2-microglobulin, which is a component of MHC class I molecules and a normal serum protein.

131.   A. T   B. T   C. T   D. T   E. T

Homogeneous or diffuse nuclear staining usually reflects antibodies to chromatin. Rim or peripheral staining patterns are most commonly indicative of antibodies to double-stranded DNA. Speckled patterns reflect the presence of antibodies to non-DNA nuclear constituents. Nucleolar pattern is most reported in systemic sclerosis. Speckled pattern is associated with extractable nuclear antigens.

4 GASTROINTESTINAL DISEASES

132. *The following statements about enteric infections are correct.*

    A. Carriers of *Salmonella typhi* with cholelithiasis often need cholecystectomy to eradicate *S. typhi*.
    B. Antidiarrhoeal drugs may increase the duration of symptoms and the risk of bacteraemia in shigellosis.
    C. *Campylobacter* enteritis usually recovers spontaneously within a week.
    D. Traveller's diarrhoea is usually caused by rotavirus.
    E. Pseudomembranous enterocolitis is caused by a toxin produced by *Clostridium difficile*.

    A........... B.......... C.......... D.......... E..........

133. *The following statements about abdominal infections are correct.*

    A. Spontaneous bacterial peritonitis usually occurs in patients with cirrhosis and ascites.
    B. Abscess formation in the peritoneum rarely requires drainage.
    C. When the peritonitis is due to a presumed gastrointestinal source, aminoglycosides should be avoided.
    D. Broad-spectrum antibiotic therapy should be initiated in uncomplicated cholecystitis.
    E. Broad-spectrum antibiotic therapy should be initiated in uncomplicated pancreatitis.

    A........... B.......... C.......... D.......... E..........

134. *Drugs contraindicated in vomiting include*

    A. prochlorperazine.
    B. intravenous metoclopramide.
    C. ondansetron.
    D. cisapride.
    E. ipecac syrup.

    A........... B.......... C.......... D.......... E..........

132. A. T   B. T   C. T   D. F   E. T

Carriers are patients who continue to excrete *S. typhi* in the stool for more than 3 months after recovery. Carriers of *S. typhi* with cholelithiasis often need cholecystectomy to eradicate the organism. Antidiarrhoeal drugs may increase the duration of symptoms and the risk of bacteraemia in shigellosis. *Campylobacter* enteritis usually recovers spontaneously within a week. Traveller's diarrhoea is usually caused by enterotoxigenic *Escherichia coli* and less often by viruses or other bacteria. Pseudomembranous enterocolitis is caused by a toxin produced by *Cl. difficile*, an anaerobe that tends to proliferate when the normal bowel flora is altered, particularly with antibiotic therapy (broad-spectrum penicillins, clindamycin and cephalosporins). Metronidazole and vancomycin are used to eradicate *Cl. difficile*.

133. A. T   B. F   C. F   D. F   E. F

Spontaneous bacterial peritonitis usually occurs in patients with cirrhosis and ascites. Abscess formation in the peritoneum usually requires percutaneous or surgical drainage. When the peritonitis is due to a presumed gastrointestinal source, the treatment includes an aminoglycoside, clindamycin or metronidazole and ampicillin or mezlocillin. Broad-spectrum antibiotic therapy should not be initiated in uncomplicated cholecystitis or pancreatitis as there is no evidence that antibiotic therapy is of benefit. It is appropriate if complicated by abscess formation, secondary peritonitis or systemic sepsis.

134. A. F   B. F   C. F   D. F   E. T

Phenothiazines including prochlorperazine are centrally acting antiemetics. Metoclopramide is a dopamine antagonist and intravenous administration is particularly useful in vomiting associated with chemotherapy and diabetic gastroparesis. Ondansetron is a $5HT_3$ antagonist used in chemotherapy-associated vomiting. Cisapride is used to enhance gastric emptying and in the treatment of vomiting. Ipecac syrup is used to induce emesis in the management of drug overdose.

135. *Causes of vomiting include*

   A. digoxin.
   B. aminophylline.
   C. increased intracranial pressure.
   D. uraemia.
   E. hypercalcaemia.

   A.......... B.......... C.......... D.......... E..........

136. *Drugs causing diarrhoea include*

   A. digitalis.
   B. quinidine.
   C. colchicine.
   D. ampicillin.
   E. opiates.

   A.......... B.......... C.......... D.......... E..........

137. *The following associations are correct.*

   A. Osmotic diarrhoea–milk of magnesia.
   B. Secretory diarrhoea–cholera.
   C. Mucosal injury–irritable bowel syndrome.
   D. Mucosal injury–Crohn's disease.
   E. Osmotic diarrhoea–lactose ingestion in lactase deficiency.

   A.......... B.......... C.......... D.......... E..........

138. *In patients with Human immunodeficiency virus (HIV)*

   A. watery diarrhoea excludes giardiasis.
   B. dysenteric symptoms are commonly associated with bacterial pathogens.
   C. anorectal symptoms should prompt investigation for venereal infections.
   D. stool examination should include acid-fast stains.
   E. small-bowel biopsy is routine for the diagnosis of diarrhoeas.

   A.......... B.......... C.......... D.......... E..........

139. *The following statements about the management of diarrhoea are correct.*

   A. Opioid agents should be used cautiously in patients with benign prostatic hypertrophy.
   B. Antiperistaltic drugs may precipitate toxic megacolon in patients with invasive bacterial infection.
   C. Somatostatin is contraindicated in patients with refractory diarrhoea due to carcinoid syndrome.
   D. Most cases of acute diarrhoea require antidiarrhoeal treatment.
   E. Non-specific antidiarrhoeals may prolong illness in *Salmonella* infections.

   A.......... B.......... C.......... D.......... E..........

135. A. T   B. T   C. T   D. T   E. T

Drugs such as digoxin and aminophylline causes vomiting. Nausea and vomiting may result from primary gastrointestinal disorders such as intestinal obstruction, viral illness (the commonest cause of vomiting in adults) and systemic illnesses, including conditions with increased intracranial pressure (such as meningitis, intracranial neoplasms), uraemia and hypercalcaemia. Pregnancy should be excluded in women of child-bearing age.

136. A. T   B. T   C. T   D. T   E. F

Digitalis, quinidine, colchicine and ampicillin cause diarrhoea. Opiates generally cause constipation.

137. A. T   B. T   C. F   D. T   E. T

Osmotic diarrhoea is caused by the accumulation of poorly absorbed solutes in the intestine and usually ameliorates with fasting. It is induced by osmotic laxatives such as milk of magnesia and ingestion of lactose in those with lactase deficiency. In cholera, the characteristic feature is secretory diarrhoea due to abnormal secretion of water and electrolytes in the lumen. This is not reduced by fasting and is caused by bacterial toxins, vasoactive intestinal peptide, gastrin, dihydroxy bile acids and fatty acids. In irritable bowel syndrome, the mucosa is intact and frequent bowel movement is due to altered intestinal motility. Mucosal injury results in diarrhoea with both osmotic and secretory components and is a feature of ulcerative colitis, Crohn's disease, coeliac sprue, lymphoma and ischaemic bowel injury.

138. A. F   B. T   C. T   D. T   E. F

Watery diarrhoea in HIV-infected patients is usually caused by giardiasis, *Mycobacterium avium-intracellulare* and cryptosporidiosis, whereas dysenteric symptoms are commonly associated with bacterial pathogens. Stool examination should include acid-fast stains; small-bowel biopsy is done only when stool examination is not conclusive. Anorectal symptoms should prompt investigation for venereal infections, particularly syphilis, gonorrhoea, chlamydiosis and herpes simplex virus.

139. A. T   B. T   C. F   D. F   E. T

Opioid agents should be used cautiously in patients with benign prostatic hypertrophy, asthma, chronic obstructive airways disease and acute angle-closure glaucoma. Non-specific antidiarrhoeals may prolong illness in *Salmonella* and *Shigella* infections and antiperistaltic drugs may precipitate toxic megacolon in patients with invasive bacterial infection. Most cases of acute diarrhoea are self-limiting and do not require treatment. Somatostatin is used in the treatment of refractory diarrhoea due to carcinoid syndrome.

140. *The following statements about constipation are correct.*

A. When constipation develops in a middle-aged or elderly individual, colon cancer should be considered.
B. Constipation is not desirable in patients with recent acute myocardial infarction.
C. Hyperparathyroidism causes constipation.
D. Emollient laxatives and mineral oil are given concurrently in the management of constipation.
E. Polyethylene glycol is useful in the management of constipation.

A............ B.......... C.......... D.......... E..........

141. *Complications of reflux oesophagitis include*

A. Barrett's oesophagus.
B. oesophageal stricture.
C. pulmonary aspiration.
D. bleeding from oesophagus.
E. hiatal hernias.

A............ B.......... C.......... D.......... E..........

142. *Medications that decrease lower oesophageal sphincter pressure include*

A. metoclopramide.
B. cisapride.
C. calcium channel blockers.
D. diazepam.
E. theophylline.

A............ B.......... C.......... D.......... E..........

143. *The following statements about peptic ulcers are correct.*

A. Most duodenal ulcers are malignant.
B. Most gastric ulcers are malignant.
C. Most peptic ulcers are associated with the presence of *Helicobacter pylori* in the stomach.
D. At least half the patients with peptic ulcers will have a recurrence within 5 years.
E. Endoscopic biopsy of gastric ulcers at the time of initial diagnosis is recommended.

A............ B.......... C.......... D.......... E..........

140.   A. T   B. T   C. T   D. F   E. T

When constipation develops in a middle-aged or elderly individual, colon cancer should be considered. Constipation is not desirable in patients with recent acute myocardial infarction or acute abdominal surgery as straining during defecation is an isometric exercise that fatigues the cardiovascular system and increases intra-abdominal pressure. Hypothyroidism, hypercalcaemia and hyperparathyroidism cause constipation. Emollient laxatives and mineral oil are not given concurrently because emollient laxatives enhance absorption of mineral oil. Polyethylene glycol, an osmotic cathartic, is useful in the management of constipation and in bowel preparation before endoscopic examination.

141.   A. T   B. T   C. T   D. T   E. F

Complications of oesophagitis include Barrett's oesophagus, oesophageal stricture, pulmonary aspiration and bleeding from oesophagus. Although hiatal hernias are often seen in patients with reflux oesophagitis, they are not a complication of the latter.

142.   A. F   B. F   C. T   D. T   E. T

Lower oesophageal sphincter pressure is reduced by alcohol, chocolate, caffeine, theophylline, diazepam, calcium channel blockers and narcotics. Metoclopramide and cisapride increase lower oesophageal sphincter pressure and are used in the management of oesophageal reflux.

143.   A. F   B. F   C. T   D. T   E. T

Duodenal ulcers are very rarely malignant whereas about 5% of gastric ulcers are malignant and hence endoscopic biopsy of gastric ulcers at the time of initial diagnosis is recommended. Gastric ulcers should be followed until completely healed to ensure they are not malignant. Most peptic ulcers are associated with the presence of H. pylori in the stomach and at least half the patients with peptic ulcers will have a recurrence within 5 years. Eradication of H. pylori has reduced the recurrence of peptic ulcer by approximately 80%. A standard regimen of oral antibiotics includes tetracycline, metronidazole and bismuth compound. The treatment of peptic ulcers also includes reduction of stomach acidity.

144. *The following statements about the mechanism of action of anti-ulcer drugs are correct.*

A. Omeprazole stimulates the hydrogen–potassium ATPase.
B. Ranitidine is an H_2-receptor agonist.
C. Sucralfate blocks acid secretion.
D. Aluminium hydroxide buffers gastric acid.
E. Clarithromycin is used to eradicate *H. pylori*.

A.......... B.......... C.......... D.......... E..........

145. *Aluminium hydroxide decreases the absorption of*

A. cimetidine.
B. omeprazole.
C. thyroxine.
D. tetracycline.
E. chlorpromazine.

A.......... B.......... C.......... D.......... E..........

146. *The following statements about the management of peptic ulcers are correct.*

A. Bland diet improves ulcer healing.
B. Late evening snacks should be avoided.
C. Cessation of cigarette smoking should be encouraged.
D. Alcohol induces recurrence of peptic ulcer.
E. Aspirin should be avoided.

A.......... B.......... C.......... D.......... E..........

147. *Side-effects of cimetidine include*

A. impotence.
B. gynaecomastia.
C. reduced sperm count.
D. impaired metabolism of warfarin.
E. confusion in the elderly.

A.......... B.......... C.......... D.......... E..........

148. *Complications of peptic ulcers include*

A. pyloric stenosis.
B. upper gastrointestinal bleeding.
C. perforation.
D. penetration into the pancreas.
E. Zollinger–Ellison syndrome.

A.......... B.......... C.......... D.......... E..........

144. A. F   B. F   C. F   D. T   E. T

Omeprazole inhibits hydrogen–potassium ATPase and profoundly decreases gastric acid secretion, ranitidine is an H_2-receptor antagonist. Sucralfate does not block acid secretion but acts locally on the surface of the mucosa and is as effective as H_2-blockers or antacids. Sucralfate reduces absorption of cimetidine, phenytoin, tetracycline, digoxin and fluoroquinolones. Aluminium hydroxide, magnesium hydroxide and calcium carbonate are antacids that buffer gastric acid. As magnesium hydroxide can cause diarrhoea it is often combined with aluminium hydroxide. Magnesium hydroxide should be avoided in renal failure. Clarithromycin or amoxycillin with omeprazole, or ranitidine with metronidazole and amoxycillin are used to eradicate *H. pylori.*

145. A. F   B. F   C. T   D. T   E. T

Aluminium hydroxide decreases absorption of thyroxine, tetracycline and chlorpromazine. It also binds phosphate in the intestine and may cause hypophosphataemia.

146. A. F   B. T   C. T   D. F   E. T

There is no evidence to indicate that bland diet improves ulcer healing or symptoms. In general, patients should avoid diets that aggravate their dyspeptic symptoms. Late evening snacks induce gastric acid production when the patient is asleep and unable to take antacids and hence snacks before going to bed should be avoided. Cigarette smoking not only increases the risk of development of peptic ulcers but also delays ulcer healing and increases the rate of ulcer recurrence. Although high doses of alcohol cause gastritis, there is no evidence that it induces recurrence of peptic ulcer.

147. A. T   B. T   C. T   D. T   E. T

Cimetidine induces reversible impotence in those on high-dose chronic therapy (as in Zollinger–Ellison syndrome) and causes gynaecomastia and reduced sperm count in patients on long-term therapy. It impairs metabolism of phenytoin, warfarin and theophyllines. It can cause confusion in the elderly, particularly when there is associated impairment of renal or hepatic function.

148. A. T   B. T   C. T   D. T   E. F

The complications of peptic ulcers are gastric outlet obstruction (including pyloric stenosis), upper gastrointestinal bleeding (haematemesis and melaena), gastric perforation, penetration into the pancreas (most often associated with ulcers in the posterior wall of the duodenal bulb) and intractability. Zollinger–Ellison syndrome is due to gastric hypersecretion caused by a gastrin-secreting islet-cell tumour of the pancreas or duodenum. This presents as a duodenal bulb ulcer or with multiple ulceration in the distal duodenum or jejunum or recurrent ulceration. Diarrhoea is the commonest symptom.

149. *The following associations are correct.*

A. Dumping syndrome–after gastrectomy.
B. Osteomalacia–Billroth II anastomosis.
C. Anaemia–after gastrectomy.
D. Diarrhoea–vagotomy.
E. Steatorrhoea–after gastrectomy.

A............   B..........   C..........   D..........   E..........

150. *Causes of gastroparesis include*

A. scleroderma.
B. diabetes mellitus.
C. hypercalcaemia.
D. hypocalcaemia.
E. anticholinergic agents.

A............   B..........   C..........   D..........   E..........

151. *Recognised features of gastrointestinal bleeding include the following.*

A. Supine hypotension suggests severe blood loss.
B. Restoration of intravascular blood volume should begin immediately.
C. Patients with cardiac or pulmonary disease may require transfusion to a higher haematocrit.
D. Melaena indicates bleeding proximal to the caecum.
E. The haemoglobin and haematocrit accurately reflect the degree of blood loss in acute bleeds.

A............   B..........   C..........   D..........   E..........

149. A. T   B. T   C. T   D. T   E. T

Dumping syndrome occurs after gastrectomy and is due to rapid gastric emptying of a large osmotic load into the upper small intestine. It manifests with vomiting and abdominal discomfort and is often accompanied by vasomotor symptoms such as sweating, palpitations and dizziness. These symptoms can be reduced by having six small meals that are high in protein and low in refined carbohydrate and by avoiding liquids during meal time. Mild steatorrhoea can occur after gastrectomy and is due to decreased intestinal transit time, resulting in diminished mixing of food with pancreatic and biliary secretions. It can also be due to bacterial overgrowth caused by afferent loop stasis. The anaemia following gastrectomy is due to the deficiency of iron, folate or vitamin B_{12}. Osteomalacia occurs in about one-third of the patients with Billroth II anastomosis and such patients should be given calcium and vitamin D supplements. Mild diarrhoea can follow vagotomy but treatable conditions such as fat malabsorption or lactase deficiency should be excluded. These patients may respond to diphenoxylate or tincture of opium therapy.

150. A. T   B. T   C. T   D. T   E. T

Causes of gastroparesis include diabetes mellitus, scleroderma, collagen vascular disorders, acute hyperglycaemia, hypercalcaemia, hypocalcaemia, tricyclic antidepressants, anticholinergic agents and narcotics. Metoclopramide and cisapride are often used in gastroparesis with mixed success.

151. A. T   B. T   C. T   D. T   E. F

Supine hypotension suggests severe blood loss, usually more than 20% of the circulatory blood volume. Postural hypotension indicates moderate blood loss, about 10–20% of the circulatory volume. Restoration of intravascular blood volume should begin immediately and vasopressors are generally avoided. Patients with cardiac or pulmonary disease may require red blood cell transfusion to a higher haematocrit to prevent ischaemia. Melaena is black tarry stools and indicates bleeding proximal to the caecum. The haemoglobin and haematocrit do not accurately reflect the degree of blood loss in acute bleeds as it takes some time for equilibration.

152. *The following statements about upper gastrointestinal bleeding are correct.*

A. Upper gastrointestinal barium radiography continues to play a major role in the initial evaluation of active bleeding even when endoscopy is available.
B. Early diagnostic upper gastrointestinal endoscopy improves mortality.
C. Arterial vasopressin controls bleeding in some patients with peptic ulcers.
D. Sclerotherapy is effective for controlling primary haemorrhage from oesophageal varices.
E. Transjugular intrahepatic portosystemic shunt is used for patients who fail sclerotherapy and have gastric variceal bleeding.

A............   B..........   C..........   D..........   E..........

153. *The following statements about coeliac sprue are correct.*

A. Patients are sensitive to a group of proteins present in rice.
B. Anti-gliadin antibodies are found in many patients.
C. Biopsy of the small intestine reveals complete absence of villi.
D. Patients commonly have secondary lactase deficiency.
E. It is associated with increased incidence of small-bowel lymphoma.

A............   B..........   C..........   D..........   E..........

154. *Recognised features of ulcerative colitis include the following.*

A. It is characterised by remissions and exacerbations.
B. The rectum is spared.
C. Patients with frequent relapses despite treatment will often require surgery.
D. Total proctocolectomy is curative.
E. Colon cancer may occur in long-standing disease.

A............   B..........   C..........   D..........   E..........

152. A. F   B. F   C. T   D. T   E. T

Upper gastrointestinal barium radiography has no role in the initial evaluation of active bleeding when endoscopy is available. Early diagnostic upper gastrointestinal endoscopy does not improve mortality but reduces length of hospital stay, transfusion requirements and the need for emergency surgery. It is useful in identifying the site of bleeding before implementing therapy such as arterial vasopressin or balloon tamponade of the oesophagus. Arterial vasopressin controls bleeding in some patients with peptic ulcers, stress ulcers and gastritis. Intravenous vasopressin is used to control variceal haemorrhage but is less effective than sclerotherapy. It should be used with great caution in patients with coronary artery disease. Sclerotherapy is effective for controlling primary haemorrhage from oesophageal varices but is associated with complications such as recurrent bleeding (in up to 50% of patients), ulceration, fever, strictures, perforations and sepsis. Transjugular intrahepatic portosystemic shunt is used for patients who fail sclerotherapy and have gastric variceal bleeding. It involves placing an expandable metal stent between the hepatic and portal veins. Portocaval and distal splenorenal shunt controls variceal bleeding in as many as 95% of patients but is associated with postoperative encephalopathy and hospital mortality.

153. A. F   B. T   C. T   D. T   E. T

Patients are sensitive to gluten, a group of proteins present in wheat, barley, rye and possibly oats. Anti–gliadin antibodies are seen in many patients. Biopsy of the small intestine reveals complete absence of villi. A gluten-free diet improves symptoms and histology in such patients. Patients commonly have secondary lactase deficiency and a lactose-free diet should be followed until the patient recovers. Sprue is associated with increased incidence of small-bowel lymphoma. Patients who deteriorate despite adhering to a gluten-free diet should be investigated for lymphoma by abdominal CT and small-bowel barium studies.

154. A. T   B. F   C. T   D. T   E. T

Ulcerative colitis is characterised by remissions and exacerbations. Patients with frequent relapses despite treatment will often require surgery. Total proctocolectomy is curative. Colon cancer may occur in long-standing disease. Patients with pancolitis have a 10% incidence of colon cancer at 10–20 years' with an additional 10% incidence for every decade thereafter.

155. *The following statements about the management of ulcerative colitis are correct.*

A. The sulphapyridine moiety in sulphasalazine is the active component.
B. Glucocorticoids are beneficial in those with moderate or severe colonic disease.
C. Immunosuppressive agents have a major role in the management of steroid-resistant colitis.
D. Elemental diets may be useful during the acute phases of the disease.
E. In toxic megacolon, total colectomy must be considered in acutely ill patients not responding to intensive medical therapy for 48 h.

A.......... B.......... C.......... D.......... E..........

156. *Recognised features of irritable bowel syndrome include*

A. loss of weight.
B. nocturnal diarrhoea.
C. alternating diarrhoea and constipation.
D. associated psychiatric symptoms.
E. lactose intolerance.

A.......... B.......... C.......... D.......... E..........

157. *Acute pancreatitis is commonly associated with*

A. excessive alcohol consumption.
B. gallstones.
C. hypercalcaemia.
D. hypertriglyceridaemia.
E. drugs.

A.......... B.......... C.......... D.......... E..........

158. *Poor prognostic factors in acute pancreatitis include*

A. elevated WBC count.
B. hyperglycaemia.
C. drop of haematocrit greater than 10%.
D. hypoxaemia
E. hypocalcaemia.

A.......... B.......... C.......... D.......... E..........

159. *Complications of acute pancreatitis include*

A. infection.
B. pseudocyst formation.
C. adult respiratory distress syndrome (ARDS).
D. acute renal failure.
E. severe haemorrhage.

A.......... B.......... C.......... D.......... E..........

155. A. F   B. T   C. F   D. T   E. T

The sulphapyridine moiety in sulphasalazine is not the active component but is responsible for most of the toxicity. The active component is 5-aminosalicylate. Mesalamine and 5-aminosalicylate lack the sulpha moiety and are associated with fewer side-effects than sulphasalazine. Side-effects of sulphasalazine include nausea, vomiting, headache, abdominal pain and hypersensitivity reactions (including fever, rash, hepatotoxicity, agranulocytosis and aplastic anaemia). Glucocorticoids are beneficial in those with moderate or severe colonic disease. Immunosuppressive agents have a limited role in the management of ulcerative colitis resistant to medical therapy. Elemental diets may be useful during the acute phases of the disease and low-roughage diets provide symptomatic relief for patients. In toxic megacolon, total colectomy must be considered in acutely ill patients not responding to intensive medical therapy for 48 h. Medical therapy for toxic megacolon includes nasogastric suction, correction of dehydration and electrolyte imbalance, broad-spectrum intravenous antibiotics and intravenous glucocorticoids.

156. A. F   B. F   C. T   D. T   E. F

Irritable bowel syndrome is characterised by long-standing crampy abdominal pain, bloating, alternating diarrhoea and constipation and excessive flatulence. Lactose intolerance should be excluded in these patients. Often the patients have associated psychiatric symptoms. Loss of weight and nocturnal diarrhoea that wakes the sleeping patient indicate an organic cause and is unlikely to be irritable bowel syndrome. Patients with irritable bowel syndrome have a stable weight and a normal physical examination.

157. A. T   B. T   C. T   D. T   E. T

Acute pancreatitis is commonly associated with excessive alcohol consumption, gallstones, hypercalcaemia, hypertriglyceridaemia and drugs.

158. A. T   B. T   C. T   D. T   E. T

Ranson's criteria are used to obtain prognosis in acute pancreatitis. Severe illness and mortality are associated with age over 55 years, blood glucose greater than $200 \, \text{mg} \, \text{dl}^{-1}$, WBC count greater than $16\,000/\text{mm}^3$, decrease in haematocrit of greater than 10%, rise in blood urea nitrogen greater than $5 \, \text{mg} \, \text{dl}^{-1}$, arterial Po_2 less than 60 mmHg, base deficit greater than $4 \, \text{mEq} \, \text{l}^{-1}$, serum calcium less than $8 \, \text{mg} \, \text{dl}^{-1}$ and estimated fluid sequestration greater than 6 l.

159. A. T   B. T   C. T   D. T   E. T

Complications of acute pancreatitis include infection (pancreatic abscess, necrosis, infected pseudocyst and aspiration pneumonia), pseudocyst formation, acute renal failure, pulmonary complications (ARDS, atelectasis, pleural effusion and pneumonia), severe haemorrhage and common bile duct or duodenal obstruction.

160. *Recognised features of chronic pancreatitis include the following.*

    A. It is usually associated with chronic alcoholism.
    B. The presence of a calcified pancreas on a plain abdominal radiograph is diagnostic of chronic pancreatitis.
    C. Many patients with chronic pancreatitis have severe pain as the major manifestation of their illness.
    D. Many patients may require supplemental insulin therapy.
    E. Oral pancreatic enzyme supplements may be beneficial for pain control in those with mild to moderate exocrine insufficiency.

    A............   B..........   C..........   D..........   E..........

161. *Non-surgical therapies for gallstones include*

    A. percutaneous instillation of contact solvents into the gallbladder.
    B. extracorporeal shock–wave lithotripsy.
    C. chenodeoxycholic acid.
    D. mesalazine.
    E. ursodeoxycholic acid.

    A............   B..........   C..........   D..........   E..........

162. *Complications of gallstones include*

    A. ascending cholangitis.
    B. pancreatitis.
    C. ileus.
    D. gallbladder empyema.
    E. gallbladder perforation.

    A............   B..........   C..........   D..........   E..........

163. *A 40-year-old male with alcoholic liver disease should be considered for hepatic transplantation when the following occur:*

    A. refractory ascites.
    B. severe hypoalbuminaemia.
    C. encephalopathy.
    D. variceal bleeding.
    E. severe coagulopathy.

    A............   B..........   C..........   D..........   E..........

160.   A. T   B. T   C. T   D. T   E. T

It is usually associated with chronic alcoholism. The presence of a calcified pancreas on a plain abdominal radiograph is diagnostic of chronic pancreatitis. Many patients with chronic pancreatitis have severe pain as the major manifestation of their illness, often requiring narcotics. Oral pancreatic enzyme supplements may be beneficial for pain control in those with mild to moderate exocrine insufficiency. Many patients have destruction of pancreatic islet cells and may require supplemental insulin therapy.

161.   A. T   B. T   C. T   D. F   E. T

Percutaneous instillation of contact solvents such as methyl-*tert*-butyl-ether into the gallbladder and extracorporeal shock-wave lithotripsy, alone or in combination, are used in the treatment of gallstones. Chenodeoxycholic acid and ursodeoxycholic acid in combination are used to treat cholesterol gallstones in those with uncomplicated biliary colic who are not eligible for surgery.

162.   A. T   B. T   C. T   D. T   E. T

Complications of gallstones include cholangitis, obstruction of the common bile duct, intestinal ileus, pancreatitis, gallbladder empyema and perforation.

163.   A. T   B. T   C. T   D. T   E. T

In chronic liver disease, hepatic transplantation should be considered when the following complications occur: refractory ascites, subacute bacterial peritonitis, encephalopathy, variceal bleeding or diminished function by the liver including low serum albumin levels or severe clotting defects. In fulminant hepatic failure, transplantation should be considered when patients develop signs of severe encephalopathy, severe clotting defects (prothrombin time > 20 s) or hypoglycaemia.

164. *The following statements are correct.*

    A. Acute liver disease refers to abnormalities present less than 6 months.
    B. Fulminant hepatic failure implies rapid progression from onset of disease to liver failure over a period of less than 4 weeks.
    C. Hepatic disorders with predominant elevations of alkaline phosphatase and 5-nucleotidase indicates absence of intrahepatic cholestasis.
    D. In haemolysis there is a predominant elevation of conjugated bilirubin.
    E. Factor VIII is synthesised in the liver.

    A.......... B.......... C.......... D.......... E..........

165. *The following statements about liver enzymes are correct.*

    A. Alanine aminotransferase is generally more sensitive than aspartate aminotransferase for detecting viral hepatitis.
    B. In alcoholic liver disease, aspartate aminotransferase is elevated in excess of alanine aminotransferase typically by a factor of two or more.
    C. Alkaline phosphatase is present in the intestine.
    D. γ-Glutamyl transpeptidase (GGT) is elevated by agents known to stimulate the hepatic microsomal mixed-function oxidase system.
    E. At the onset of acute liver disease, serum albumin levels are almost always low.

    A.......... B.......... C.......... D.......... E..........

166. *The following statements about viral hepatitis are correct.*

    A. Due to faecal shedding of hepatitis A virus, precautions to prevent faeco-oral contamination must be taken in the first 2–3 weeks of the illness.
    B. Hepatitis B surface antigen (HBsAg) is detectable in serum in almost all cases of acute and chronic hepatitis B virus infection.
    C. Hepatitis B core antigen (HBcAg) is usually detected in serum when there is active viral replication.
    D. Patients with active hepatitis B virus infection should avoid sharing toothbrushes or razors with other household members.
    E. HBsAg is present in other body fluids such as saliva and semen.

    A.......... B.......... C.......... D.......... E..........

167. *The following statements are correct.*

    A. The presence of hepatitis C virus antibody confers long-term immunity from subsequent infection by the virus.
    B. Sexual transmission occurs more frequently when the patient carries both HIV and hepatitis C virus.
    C. Hepatitis D virus requires the presence of hepatitis B virus for infection and replication to occur.
    D. Transmission of hepatitis E virus closely resembles that of hepatitis A virus.
    E. Transmission and isolation recommendations for non-A, non-B hepatitis virus infections are similar to those for hepatitis C virus.

    A.......... B.......... C.......... D.......... E..........

164.   A. T   B. T   C. F   D. F   E. F

Acute liver disease refers to abnormalities present less than 6 months whereas chronic liver disease refers to abnormalities existing for over 6 months. Fulminant hepatic failure implies rapid progression from onset of disease to liver failure over a period of less than 4 weeks. Hepatic disorders with predominant elevations of alkaline phosphatase and 5-nucleotidase indicates cholestasis. In haemolysis there is a predominant elevation of unconjugated bilirubin. Unconjugated bilirubin occurs also in ineffective erythropoiesis, Gilbert's syndrome, Crigler–Najjar syndrome or reduced hepatic bilirubin uptake (as in portosystemic shunting and heart failure). Conjugated bilirubin is elevated in hepatocellular damage or obstruction to the biliary tract. Factor VIII is the only coagulation factor not synthesised in the liver. Synthesis of factors II, VII, IX and X depends on the presence of vitamin K. Hence prolongation of prothrombin time (which determines the function of factors II, V, VII and X) indicates either a deficiency of vitamin K or impaired hepatic synthesis. The former can be excluded if prothrombin time returns to normal after administration of vitamin K.

165.   A. T   B. T   C. T   D. T   E. F

Alanine aminotransferase is generally more sensitive than aspartate aminotransferase for detecting viral hepatitis. In alcoholic liver disease, aspartate aminotransferase is elevated in excess of alanine aminotransferase typically by a factor of two or more. Alkaline phosphatase is present in the intestine, bone and liver. GGT is elevated by agents known to stimulate the hepatic microsomal mixed-function oxidase system (e.g. alcohol, phenytoin or barbiturates). In acute liver disease, serum albumin levels are frequently normal because the half-life of albumin is about 3 weeks.

166.   A. T   B. T   C. F   D. T   E. T

Hepatitis A virus spreads by the faeco-oral route and hence precautions must be taken in the first 2–3 weeks of the illness to prevent this from occurring. HBsAg is detectable in serum in almost all cases of acute and chronic hepatitis B virus infection. HBcAg does not freely circulate but is present in liver cells during replication of the hepatitis B virus. HBeAg is a component of HBcAg and circulates in the serum during active viral replication. Patients with active hepatitis B virus infection should avoid sharing toothbrushes or razors with other household members. HBsAg is present in other body fluids such as saliva and semen.

167.   A. F   B. T   C. T   D. T   E. T

The presence of hepatitis C virus antibody does not confer immunity from subsequent infection by the virus. Sexual transmission occurs more frequently when the patient carries both HIV and hepatitis C virus. Hepatitis D virus requires the presence of hepatitis B virus for infection and replication to occur. Transmission of hepatitis E virus closely resembles that of hepatitis A virus. Transmission and isolation recommendations for non-A, non-B hepatitis virus infections are similar to those for hepatitis C virus.

168. *The following statements about the management of viral hepatitis are correct.*

   A. Pre-exposure prophylaxis for hepatitis A with immune serum globulin should be given to travellers to endemic areas.
   B. Universal vaccination for hepatitis B is recommended for all infants.
   C. Fat intake should be restricted during the course of the illness.
   D. Management of acute hepatitis is predominantly performed on an outpatient basis.
   E. In patients undergoing haemodialysis, plasma-derived hepatitis B vaccination is recommended.

   A.......... B.......... C.......... D.......... E..........

169. *A 30-year-old woman with acute paracetamol overdose has jaundice, encephalopathy and prolonged prothrombin time. The following statements are correct.*

   A. Caloric intake should be maintained with intravenous dextrose-containing fluids.
   B. Prophylactic fresh frozen plasma should be administered.
   C. Glucocorticoids usually have a dramatic effect in those with associated cerebral oedema.
   D. If she lapses into coma unresponsive to stimuli, hepatic transplantation should be considered.
   E. H_2-receptor antagonists should be avoided.

   A.......... B.......... C.......... D.......... E..........

170. *The following statements about chronic viral hepatitis are correct.*

   A. The carrier state is characterised by elevated hepatic enzymes but no inflammation on biopsy.
   B. Chronic persistent hepatitis is characterised by the presence of chronic inflammation involving both the portal tracts and the periportal parenchyma.
   C. Chronic active hepatitis is characterised by the presence of chronic inflammation limited to the portal tracts.
   D. Cirrhosis is characterised by the presence of severe fibrosis and regenerating nodules.
   E. In patients with chronic hepatitis B, interferon-α therapy can result in remission in almost all patients.

   A.......... B.......... C.......... D.......... E..........

171. *Poor prognostic factors in acute alcoholic hepatitis include*

   A. prolongation of prothrombin time that does not normalise with vitamin K.
   B. elevated total bilirubin.
   C. leucocytosis.
   D. elevated blood urea nitrogen.
   E. elevated serum creatinine.

   A.......... B.......... C.......... D.......... E..........

168.   A. T   B. T   C. F   D. T   E. T

Pre-exposure prophylaxis for hepatitis A with immune serum globulin should be given to travellers to endemic areas. Universal vaccination for hepatitis B is recommended for all infants, with recombinant hepatitis B virus being administered intramuscularly. All infants of hepatitis B-infected mothers should receive hepatitis B vaccinations and hepatitis B immune globulin within 12 h of birth. In patients undergoing haemodialysis, plasma-derived hepatitis B vaccination is recommended. Diet therapy has no major role in the management of acute hepatitis and fat intake is restricted in individuals with nausea, vomiting or diarrhoea. Management of acute hepatitis is predominantly performed on an outpatient basis.

169.   A. T   B. F   C. F   D. T   E. F

This patient has fulminant hepatic failure. Caloric intake should be maintained with intravenous dextrose-containing fluids. Prophylactic fresh frozen plasma should be avoided as it may lead to volume overload and make assessment of residual synthetic function of the liver difficult. Glucocorticoids usually have almost no effect in those with associated cerebral oedema. If she lapses into coma unresponsive to stimuli, hepatic transplantation should be considered. H_2-receptor antagonists and anatacids should be used to keep gastric pH above 5 to prevent upper gastrointestinal bleeds.

170.   A. F   B. F   C. F   D. T   E. F

The carrier state is characterised by normal hepatic enzymes and no inflammation on biopsy but persistent circulating viral particles. Chronic persistent hepatitis is characterised by the presence of chronic inflammation limited to the portal tracts. Chronic active hepatitis is characterised by the presence of chronic inflammation involving both the portal tracts and the periportal parenchyma. Cirrhosis is characterised by the presence of severe fibrosis and regenerating nodules. In patients with chronic hepatitis B, interferon-α therapy administered for about 4 months can result in histological and biochemical remission in about one-third of patients.

171.   A. T   B. T   C. T   D. T   E. T

Poor prognostic factors include prolongation of prothrombin time that does not normalise with vitamin K, elevated total bilirubin, leucocytosis, elevated blood urea nitrogen and elevated serum creatinine.

172. *Recognised features of primary biliary cirrhosis include*

   A. absence of pruritus.
   B. absence of anti-mitochondrial antibodies.
   C. elevated bile acids.
   D. low levels of IgM.
   E. spontaneous fractures.

   A.......... B.......... C.......... D.......... E..........

173. *Recognised features of primary sclerosing cholangitis include the following*

   A. It is more common in middle-aged women.
   B. Patients are at high risk of developing cholangiosarcoma.
   C. Hepatic transplantation is contraindicated in recurrent cholangitis.
   D. There is a frequent association with inflammatory bowel disease.
   E. Ursodeoxycholic acid is the treatment of choice during acute episodes.

   A.......... B.......... C.......... D.......... E..........

174. *Recognised features of Wilson's disease include*

   A. dominant inheritance.
   B. neuropsychiatric symptoms.
   C. high serum caeruloplasmin levels.
   D. low hepatic copper levels.
   E. Kayser–Fleischer ring.

   A.......... B.......... C.......... D.......... E..........

175. *Recognised features of haemochromatosis include*

   A. low serum α_1-antitrypsin levels.
   B. cardiomyopathy.
   C. diabetes.
   D. high transferrin saturation.
   E. increased risk for development of hepatomas despite therapy.

   A.......... B.......... C.......... D.......... E..........

176. *Recognised features of Budd–Chiari syndrome include the following:*

   A. ascites.
   B. enlargement of the caudate lobe.
   C. increased venous thrombosis.
   D. it is due to hepatic arterial occlusion.
   E. it is associated with lymphoreticular malignancies.

   A.......... B.......... C.......... D.......... E..........

172.   A. F   B. F   C. T   D. F   E. T

Primary biliary cirrhosis is characteristically seen in middle-aged women and has a variable natural history with some patients being asymptomatic for several years. Pruritus is the most common symptom and can be troublesome. Cholestyramine is given for pruritus, but should not be given concurrently with vitamins or other medications as it may impair their absorption. Typical clinical features include elevated levels of alkaline phosphatase, bile acids, cholesterol and IgM. Anti-mitochondrial antibodies are elevated in 95% of patients with primary biliary cirrhosis. Spontaneous fractures due to osteoporosis and osteomalacia can occur.

173.   A. F   B. T   C. F   D. T   E. F

Primary sclerosing cholangitis is more common in middle-aged men and those patients are at high risk of developing cholangiosarcoma. There is a frequent association with inflammatory bowel disease. No specific therapy has proved successful and ursodeoxycholic acid, cyclosporin and methotrexate remain experimental modalities of treatment. Hepatic transplantation should be considered in recurrent cholangitis or advanced disease.

174.   A. F   B. T   C. F   D. F   E. T

Wilson's disease is inherited recessively and is characterised by copper overload in the liver, resulting in hepatic dysfunction and neuropsychiatric symptoms. The Kayser–Fleischer ring is a deposit of copper along Descemet's membrane of the cornea. Copper levels are elevated, serum caeruloplasmin is low and urinary copper is elevated. Diagnosis is confirmed by quantitative liver biopsy showing high copper. Treatment involves copper chelating agents such as penicillamine and trientine. Hepatic transplantation should be considered in those not responding to chelation therapy or in fulminant hepatic failure.

175.   A. F   B. T   C. T   D. T   E. T

Haemochromatosis is a recessively inherited disorder characterised by elevated serum iron, high transferrin saturation and elevated hepatic tissue iron levels. Clinical features include slate-coloured greyish-blue pigmentation, diabetes mellitus, cardiomyopathy, chondrocalcinosis, arthritis and hepatic dysfunction. Treatment consists of regular phlebotomy. The risk for development of hepatoma persists despite therapy.

176.   A. T   B. T   C. T   D. F   E. T

Budd–Chiari syndrome is due to thrombosis of the hepatic vein and features include ascites and hepatomegaly, particularly the caudate lobe. It is a hypercoagulable state and is associated with lymphoreticular malignancies.

177. *The following statements about the management of complications of hepatic insufficiency are correct.*

   A. Vegetable-derived protein diets are better tolerated in patients with encephalopathy than diets containing animal protein.
   B. Lactulose is used in the management of encephalopathy.
   C. Diuretic dose for treatment of ascites should be escalated in patients with increasing serum creatinine levels in order to maintain renal perfusion.
   D. Empirical antibiotic therapy should be avoided in suspected cases of bacterial peritonitis.
   E. Water restriction is routine in the management of ascites.

   A.......... B.......... C.......... D.......... E..........

178. *The following statements about viral hepatitis during pregnancy are correct.*

   A. Hepatitis B during pregnancy increases prematurity.
   B. At time of delivery, HBeAg-positive mothers transmit the disease less frequently than HBsAg-positive and HBeAg-negative mothers.
   C. Infants born to mothers with hepatitis B should be treated with both hepatitis B immune globulin and hepatitis B vaccine.
   D. There is a very high risk of transmission of hepatitis A to the neonate.
   E. Hepatitis A worsens during pregnancy.

   A.......... B.......... C.......... D.......... E..........

179. *Swallowing involves all of the following.*

   A. involuntary movement of the tongue against the hard palate.
   B. voluntary relaxation of the upper oesophageal sphincter.
   C. closure of the glottis.
   D. persistalsis of the oesophagus.
   E. activation of the brainstem.

   A.......... B.......... C.......... D.......... E..........

180. *The stomach secretes*

   A. chyme.
   B. hydrochloric acid.
   C. gastrin.
   D. pepsin.
   E. amylase.

   A.......... B.......... C.......... D.......... E..........

177.   A. T   B. T   C. F   D. F   E. F

Vegetable-derived protein diets are better tolerated in patients with encephalopathy than diets containing animal protein. Lactulose is used in the management of encephalopathy. Diuretic dose for treatment of ascites should not be increased in patients with increasing serum creatinine levels to maintain renal perfusion. Empirical antibiotic therapy should be initiated in suspected cases of bacterial peritonitis, after ascitic and blood cultures have been taken. Salt and not water restriction is routine in the management of ascites. Water or fluid restriction is limited to those with severe hyponatraemia.

178.   A. T   B. F   C. T   D. F   E. F

Hepatitis B during pregnancy increases prematurity. At time of delivery, HBeAg-positive mothers transmit the disease more frequently than HBsAg-positive and HBeAg-negative mothers. Infants born to mothers with hepatitis B should be treated with both hepatitis B immune globulin and hepatitis B vaccine. The risk of transmission of hepatitis A to the neonate is low. Hepatitis A does not worsen during pregnancy.

179.   A. F   B. F   C. T   D. T   E. T

The process of deglutition or swallowing involves activation of the pharyngeal region of the brainstem, closure of the glottis, involuntary relaxation of the upper oesophageal sphincter and peristalsis of the oesophagus.

180.   A. F   B. T   C. T   D. T   E. F

Amylase is secreted by the salivary glands and pancreas whereas chyme is the product of digestion. Gastrin, hydrochloric acid and pepsin are secreted by the stomach.

181. *The following statements about cholecystokinin are correct.*

A. It inhibits secretion of pancreatic enzymes.
B. It promotes gastric emptying.
C. It regulates gallbladder contraction.
D. It is released mainly in response to proteins and fat in chyme.
E. It plays a major role in regulating insulin secretion.

A...........   B..........   C..........   D..........   E..........

181.   A. T   B. F   C. F   D. T   E. F

Cholecystokinin is released mainly in response to the presence of fat and protein in chyme. It inhibits gastric emptying, stimulates secretion of pancreatic enzymes and regulates gallbladder contraction.

5 HAEMATOLOGY AND ONCOLOGY

182. A 6-year-old boy complained of tiredness and examination showed several bruises. Haematology revealed haemoglobin $5.7\,g\,dl^{-1}$, haematocrit 20%, mean corpuscular volume (MCV) 80fl, mean corpuscular haemoglobin (MCH) 22pg, erythrocyte sedimentation rate (ESR) 80mm in first hour, reticulocytes 0.1%, platelets $9 \times 10^9/l$, WBC count is $8.7 \times 10^9/l$, neutrophils 12%, lymphocytes 40% and blast cells 51%. Blood smear showed thrombocytopenia and negligible cytoplasm.

   A. This patient has chronic lymphatic leukaemia.
   B. Children with this condition respond poorly to treatment.
   C. Chemotherapy should be avoided in this condition.
   D. This condition has a propensity to involve the CNS.
   E. Adults having this condition respond dramatically to treatment.

   A........... B.......... C.......... D.......... E..........

183. A 70-year-old man presented with recurrent chest infections. Haematology revealed haemoglobin $12\,g\,dl^{-1}$, packed cell volume (PCV) 40%, MCV 85fl, MCH 30pg, MCH concentration (MCHC) $30\,g\,dl^{-1}$, ESR 70mm in first hour, reticulocytes 1.5%, platelets $94 \times 10^9/l$, WBC count $21 \times 10^9/l$, neutrophils 34% and lymphocytes 60%. Blood smear showed small mature lymphocytes. The following statements are correct.

   A. This patient has generalised lymphadenopathy.
   B. The blood smear excludes chronic lymphatic leukaemia.
   C. In this patient Coombs' test is positive if haemolysis is occurring.
   D. This disease almost always has a fulminant course after diagnosis.
   E. Chlorambucil is the chemotherapeutic agent most often used.

   A........... B.......... C.......... D.......... E..........

184. A 65-year-old women had mass in the abdomen. Haematology revealed haemoglobin $10\,g\,dl^{-1}$, PCV 29%, MCV 80fl, MCH 27pg, MCHC $35\,g\,dl^{-1}$, ESR 34mm in first hour, reticulocytes 1.5%, platelets $350 \times 10^9/l$, WBC count $22 \times 10^9/l$, neutrophils 30%, lymphocytes 40%, blasts 3%, myelocytes 10% and metamyelocytes 10%, basophils 6%. The following statements are correct.

   A. This patient has chronic myeloid leukaemia.
   B. The majority of patients with this condition die within 5 years of diagnosis.
   C. Busulphan is used to control WBC count.
   D. Bone marrow transplantation is curative.
   E. Occasionally this condition transforms to myelofibrosis.

   A........... B.......... C.......... D.......... E..........

182. A. F   B. F   C. F   D. T   E. F

This child has acute lymphoblastic leukaemia (ALL). Predominantly a disease of children, ALL is also potentially curable. Overall 90% of children respond to treatment and 50–60% are cured. The results in adults are not as good, with only approximately 30% being cured. Cyclical combination chemotherapy comprising vincristine, prednisolone and an anthracycline such as doxorubicin forms the basis of most treatment regimens. This condition has a propensity to involve the CNS; thus treatment also includes prophylactic intrathecal drugs with or without prophylactic radiation to the cranium.

183. A. T   B. F   C. T   D. F   E. T

This patient has chronic lymphatic leukaemia. Patient has symptoms of anaemia due to haemolysis, recurrent infections due to neutropenia with or without reduced immunoglobulin levels. Clinical signs include anaemia, generalised lymph node enlargement and enlarged liver with or without splenomegaly. Coombs' test is positive if haemolysis is occurring. A proportion of the patients remain asymptomatic and never need any treatment, dying of an unrelated cause; in the remainder the disease can usually be kept under control for 9–10 years, infection being the predominant cause of death. There is no advantage to starting treatment before there is a clinical indication, e.g. anaemia, recurrent infections, bleeding, bulky lymphadenopathy or increasing splenomegaly. Chlorambucil is most often used.

184. A. T   B. T   C. T   D. T   E. T

This patient has chronic myeloid leukaemia. The majority of patients with this condition die within 5 years of diagnosis. Busulphan is used to control WBC count and reduce the size of the spleen. Bone marrow transplantation is curative but is limited by age of the patient, donor availability and mortality and morbidity of the transplant procedure. Occasionally this condition transforms to myelofibrosis, death ensuing from bone marrow failure.

185. *Haematological manifestations of pre-eclampsia include*

   A. thrombocythaemia.
   B. elevated LDH.
   C. microangiopathic haemolytic anaemia.
   D. polycythaemia.
   E. disseminated intravascular coagulation (DIC).

   A............ B........... C........... D........... E...........

186. *The following statements about the coagulation cascade are correct.*

   A. Platelet aggregation is the initial step in the coagulation cascade.
   B. The extrinsic pathway requires exposure of blood to tissue factor.
   C. Tissue factor is normally present in blood cells and intact endothelium.
   D. The molecular factors that trigger the intrinsic pathway are poorly understood.
   E. Deficiency of factor XII causes clinical bleeding.

   A............ B........... C........... D........... E...........

187. *The following associations between the dose and effects of aspirin are correct.*

   A. Analgesic effect: 80–325 mg daily.
   B. Antiplatelet effect: 650 mg every 3–4 h.
   C. Anti-inflammatory effect: 650 mg every 3–4 h.
   D. Keratolytic effect: 650 mg orally once a day.
   E. Anti-pyretic effect: 4–8 g daily.

   A............ B........... C........... D........... E...........

188. *The following statements about aspirin used for antiplatelet therapy are correct.*

   A. Aspirin causes reversible inactivation of cyclooxygenase in circulating platelets.
   B. Aspirin should be given every day for full benefit.
   C. Adding aspirin to thrombolytic therapy increases the risk of major bleeds.
   D. Aspirin at a dose of $1\,mg\,kg^{-1}$ daily is as effective as higher doses in the majority of patients at risk.
   E. Low-dose aspirin (100 mg daily) and anticoagulants are more effective than anticoagulants alone in reducing thromboembolic complications of prosthetic heart valves.

   A............ B........... C........... D........... E...........

185.   A. F   B. T   C. T   D. F   E. T

Pre-eclampsia is a disease of late pregnancy in which hypertension is associated with renal, hepatic, neurological and haematological involvement. Haematological manifestations include thrombocytopenia with elevated LDH, microangiopathic haemolytic anaemia and (DIC). The latter can cause an elevation of fibrin degradation products (FDPs) and a reduction in fibrinogen.

186.   A. F   B. T   C. F   D. T   E. F

Primary haemostasis including platelet adherence to the subendothelial matrix and platelet aggregation are not part of the coagulation cascade. Platelet adherence requires von Willebrand factor. Platelet aggregation results in a haemostatic platelet plug that releases thromboxane A_2, which causes vasoconstriction. The coagulation cascade has an intrinsic and an extrinsic pathway that together result in the formation of a fibrin clot by the generation of thrombin from prothrombin. Thrombin cleaves fibrinogen to generate fibrin; in addition, thrombin helps in the activation of factors V, VIII and XIII. The extrinsic pathway requires exposure of blood to tissue factor. Tissue factor is normally absent in blood cells and intact endothelium but is present in most extravascular tissues. The molecular factors that trigger the intrinsic pathway are poorly understood. Deficiencies of intrinsic factors such as factor XII, high molecular weight kininogen and prekallikrein do not cause clinical bleeding despite the fact that they prolong the activated partial thrombinplastin time (aPTT) like other intrinsic factors.

187.   A. F   B. F   C. F   D. F   E. T

Aspirin has antipyretic and analgesic effects in doses of 4–8 g daily, which are used in rheumatic fever. At intermediate doses of 650 mg every 3–4 h it has analgesic and antipyretic effects but not an anti-inflammatory effect. At the lowest dosage of 80–325 mg daily it exerts only an antiplatelet effect. Salicylates applied locally can dissolve corns from toes, i.e. a keratolytic effect. Aspirin also has a uricosuric effect and can kill bacteria *in vitro*, i.e. an antiseptic effect.

188.   A. F   B. T   C. F   D. T   E. T

Although aspirin causes irreversible inactivation of cyclooxygenase in circulating platelets, it should be given daily because 10% of the platelets are renewed every day and only 10% of the non-aspirin-treated platelets are sufficient to generate thromboxane A_2-dependent platelet aggregation. Although aspirin at a dose of 1 mg kg^{-1} daily is as effective as higher doses in the majority of patients at risk, some patients require as much as 325 mg daily due to limited bioavailability. When added to thrombolytic therapy aspirin does not increase the risk of major bleeds, whereas in patients with prosthetic heart valves doses of aspirin greater than 100 mg daily increase the risk of gastrointestinal bleeding. Low-dose aspirin (100 mg daily) and anticoagulants are more effective than anticoagulants alone in reducing thromboembolic complications of prosthetic heart valves.

189. *The following statements about intravenous thrombolytic therapy during acute myocardial infarction are correct.*

   A. It salvages left ventricular function, particularly when the anterior wall is involved.
   B. It recanalises the artery in 75% of the occluded coronary arteries.
   C. The improvements in mortality are equivalent for streptokinase, tissue plasminogen activator (t-PA) and anisoylated plasminogen streptokinase activator complex (APSAC).
   D. The most dreaded complication is intracranial bleeding.
   E. The addition of heparin significantly increases the risk of major bleeding.

   A.......... B.......... C.......... D.......... E..........

190. *The following statements about fibrinolysis are correct.*

   A. Fibrin is degraded by plasmin.
   B. Plasmin is converted to plasminogen by t-PA.
   C. Plasminogen may be activated by urokinase.
   D. FDPs can bind to fibrin monomers and inhibit coagulation.
   E. Circulating plasminogen activator inhibitors serve to promote fibrinolysis.

   A.......... B.......... C.......... D.......... E..........

191. *The following statements are correct.*

   A. Prostacyclin (PGI$_2$) promotes platelet aggregation.
   B. Heparin inhibits the action of antithrombin III.
   C. Thrombomodulin inhibits the activation of protein C by thrombin.
   D. In the presence of protein S, activated protein C further inhibits coagulation.
   E. Antithrombin III inhibits activated factors IX, X and XI.

   A.......... B.......... C.......... D.......... E..........

189.   A. T   B. T   C. T   D. T   E. T

Intravenous thrombolytic therapy recanalises about 75% of occluded coronary
arteries and controlled trials have shown that it salvages left ventricular function
in acute myocardial infarction (MI), particularly when the anterior wall is
involved and patients receive therapy early. Preservation in left ventricular
function and improvements in mortality are equivalent for streptokinase, t-PA
and APSAC, although t-PA causes less systemic fibrinogenolysis due to fibrin-
dependent generation of plasmin. One explanation for this difference is the rapid
clearance of t-PA; consequently thrombolysis is rapidly diminishing and early
reocclusion is enhanced. In contrast, streptokinase and APSAC produce systemic
fibrinogenolysis and the levels of FDPs inhibit both platelet function and fibrin
formation. The most dreaded complication is intracranial bleeding. Clinical
bleeding is equivalent for all three thrombolytic agents despite the fibrin
specificity of t-PA. Addition of heparin increases the risk of major bleeding
following thrombolytic therapy.

190.   A. T   B. F   C. T   D. T   E. F

Plasmin degrades fibrin by proteolysis. Plasmin is generated from fibrin-bound
plasminogen by the action of t-PA. Other enzymes that activate plasminogen
include urokinase (a urinary tract enzyme) and streptokinase (produced by β-
haemolytic streptococci). Circulating plasminogen activator inhibitors serve to
inhibit fibrinolysis. FDPs can bind to fibrin monomers and inhibit coagulation.
FDPs are produced by the action of plasmin on fibrinogen or fibrin.

191.   A. F   B. F   C. F   D. T   E. T

PGI_2 inhibits platelet aggregation. PGI_2 is synthesised by endothelial cells and
can also promote vasodilatation. Heparin promotes the action of antithrombin
III. Antithrombin III inhibits the actions of activated factors II (i.e. thrombin),
IX, X and XI. It does so by forming irreversible complexes with these proteases.
Thrombomodulin promotes the activation of protein C by thrombin and
inhibits the procoagulant activities of thrombin. In the presence of protein S,
activated protein C further inhibits coagulation by degrading activated factors V
and VIII.

192. *The following statements about the laboratory evaluation of bleeding disorders are correct.*

A. Normally there are about 10–20 platelets per oil immersion field.
B. Fragmented erythrocytes exclude microangiopathy.
C. Pseudothrombocytopenia is due to sodium citrate-induced platelet clumping.
D. Aspirin may prolong bleeding time for up to 1 week following ingestion.
E. Platelet aggregometry is usually useful in the evaluation of acquired bleeding disorders.

A............   B...........   C...........   D...........   E...........

193. *The following statements about von Willebrand factor (vWF) are correct.*

A. It is synthesised by megakaryocytes.
B. It is required for platelet adhesion.
C. It diminishes the half-life of factor VIII.
D. Ristocetin cofactor activity is increased in von Willebrand's disease.
E. The measurement of vWF antigen is useful in the subclassification of von Willebrand's disease.

A............   B...........   C...........   D...........   E...........

194. *The following statements about the evaluation of coagulation factor activity are correct.*

A. The distinction between a coagulation factor deficiency and an acquired inhibitor can be made by repeating the abnormal coagulation test using a 50 : 50 mixture of normal plasma with patient's plasma.
B. Prothrombin time is the clotting time measured after addition of tissue thromboplastin and phospholipids to recalcified plasma.
C. The aPTT time is the clotting time measured after addition of phospholipid to recalcified plasma that has been incubated with particulate material to initiate activation of the contact system.
D. Thrombin time is prolonged in DIC.
E. The presence of a lupus anticoagulant can be confirmed by comparing the clotting time of the patient's plasma with control plasma in the presence of a dilute concentration of phospholipids.

A............   B...........   C...........   D...........   E...........

192. A. T   B. F   C. F   D. T   E. F

Normally there are about 10–20 platelets per oil immersion field. Fragmented erythrocytes suggest microangiopathic disorders such as haemolytic–uraemic syndrome, DIC or thrombotic thrombocytopenic purpura. Pseudothrombocytopenia is due to EDTA (ethylenediaminetetraacetic acid)-induced platelet clumping. In such instances the peripheral blood smear should be examined and the platelet count repeated using a blood sample with sodium citrate as the anticoagulant. Bleeding time is a functional test of haemostasis; aspirin may prolong bleeding time for up to 1 week following ingestion. Prolonged bleeding time is seen in thrombocytopenia, qualitative platelet abnormalities, von Willebrand's disease and vascular disorders such as Cushing's syndrome and connective tissue disorders including vasculitis. Platelet aggregometry is usually not useful in evaluation of acquired bleeding abnormalities but is used to classify congenital platelet disorders such as Bernard–Soulier syndrome and Glanzmann's thrombasthenia.

193. A. T   B. T   C. F   D. F   E. T

vWF is synthesised by the endothelium and megakaryocytes. Evaluation of vWF should be considered in patients with a prolonged bleeding time despite a normal platelet count and no obvious cause of platelet dysfunction (such as antiplatelet drugs). vWF forms multimers comprising two to more than 40 subunits. It is required for normal platelet adhesion and also prolongs the half-life of factor VIII. Ristocetin cofactor activity is reduced in most patients with von Willebrand's disease and in paraproteinaemias with elevated protein. It is measured *in vitro*, by determining the ability of ristocetin to allow vWF to interact with platelet glycoprotein Ib. vWF antigen, also referred to as factor VIII-related antigen, is used in the subclassification of von Willebrand's disease.

194. A. T   B. T   C. T   D. T   E. T

The distinction between a coagulation factor deficiency and an acquired inhibitor can be made by repeating the abnormal coagulation test using a 50 : 50 mixture of normal plasma with patient's plasma. Prothrombin time is the clotting time measured after addition of tissue thromboplastin and phospholipids to recalcified plasma. Prothrombin time is standardised using the international normalised ratio (INR) and measures the activity of the extrinsic and common pathways. The aPTT (used to assess the intrinsic pathway) is the clotting time measured after addition of phospholipid to recalcified plasma that has been incubated with particulate material to initiate activation of the contact system. Thrombin time is prolonged in DIC and other disorders of fibrinogen. Lupus anticoagulant was initially described in patients with systemic lupus erythematosus and was found to interfere with coagulation assays *in vitro* by binding to phospholipids. The presence of a lupus anticoagulant can be confirmed by comparing the clotting time of the patient's plasma with control plasma in the presence of a dilute concentration of phospholipids. *In vivo*, lupus anticoagulant is associated with venous and arterial thrombosis.

195. *A 35-year-old female patient has a platelet count of $70 \times 10^9/l$. The following statements are correct*

   A. Normal or increased megakaryocytes in the bone marrow aspirate suggests increased platelet destruction.
   B. Intramuscular injections should be avoided.
   C. Dental floss can safely be used.
   D. Prothombin time is prolonged.
   E. This blood picture occurs in about 5–10% of pregnancies.

   A...........   B..........   C..........   D..........   E..........

196. *The associations between the following drugs and their predominant mechanism of thrombocytopenia are correct.*

   A. Thiazides: increased platelet destruction.
   B. Quinine: decreased platelet production.
   C. Ethanol: decreased platelet production.
   D. Penicillin: decreased platelet production.
   E. Chemotherapeutic agents: increased platelet destruction.

   A...........   B..........   C..........   D..........   E..........

197. *A 25-year-old female was diagnosed as having idiopathic thrombocytopenic purpura. The following statements are correct.*

   A. It can occur in a previously healthy individual.
   B. It is associated with lymphomas.
   C. It usually remits in chronic cases.
   D. When splenectomy is contemplated, pneumococcal vaccine should be administered before the procedure.
   E. Platelet transfusions are useful in the routine management.

   A...........   B..........   C..........   D..........   E..........

198. *Recognised features of thrombotic thrombocytopenic purpura (TTP) include*

   A. schistocytes on peripheral blood smear.
   B. renal dysfunction.
   C. depressed reticulocyte count.
   D. neurological manifestations.
   E. absence of laboratory evidence of DIC.

   A...........   B..........   C..........   D..........   E..........

199. *The following are X-linked disorders:*

   A. von Willebrand's disease.
   B. factor VIII deficiency.
   C. factor IX deficiency.
   D. vitamin K deficiency.
   E. DIC.

   A...........   B..........   C..........   D..........   E..........

195. A. T   B. T   C. F   D. F   E. T

Thrombocytopenia could be due to decreased platelet production or increased platelet destruction. Normal or increased megakaryocytes in the bone marrow aspirate suggests increased platelet destruction. Intramuscular injections, use of dental floss, metal razors or any trauma should be avoided. Prothrombin time is not affected, although bleeding time may be prolonged. Thrombocytopenia occurs in about 5–10% of pregnancies without significant maternal or fetal morbidity.

196. A. F   B. F   C. T   D. F   E. F

Drugs that decrease platelet production include ethanol, thiazides, trimethoprim–sulphamethoxazole, oestrogens and chemotherapeutic agents. Immune destruction of platelets is caused by penicillin, quinine, quinidine, heparin, gold salts, sulphonamides and rifampicin. Usually platelet counts are restored when the offending drug is withdrawn. In recalcitrant cases prednisolone has been used to treat thrombocytopenia.

197. A. T   B. T   C. F   D. T   E. F

Idiopathic thrombocytopenic purpura can occur in previously healthy individuals. It is associated with lymphomas, chronic lymphatic leukaemia and systemic lupus erythematosus. It usually resolves in acute cases but rarely remits in chronic cases. Management of chronic cases includes steroids, splenectomy, immunosuppressive agents, danazol and immune globulins. When splenectomy is contemplated, pneumococcal vaccine should be administered before the procedure. Platelet transfusions are of limited use because there is rapid destruction of the transfused platelets. It may be useful in those with life-threatening bleeding.

198. A. T   B. T   C. F   D. T   E. T

Features of TTP include schistocytes on peripheral blood smear, renal dysfunction, elevated reticulocyte count and lactic dehydrogenase, neurological manifestations and absence of laboratory evidence of DIC. A closely related disorder is haemolytic–uraemic syndrome. TTP is a medical emergency and initial management includes plasmapheresis using fresh frozen plasma. Refractory cases respond to splenectomy.

199. A. F   B. T   C. T   D. F   E. T

Both haemophilia A (factor VIII deficiency) and haemophilia B (factor IX deficiency) are X-linked disorders, unlike von Willebrand's disease. Vitamin K deficiency and DIC are acquired disorders. Vitamin K deficiency is associated with warfarin anticoagulants, biliary tract obstruction, malabsorption, nutritional deficiency and antibiotic therapy. Vitamin K is a necessary cofactor for the γ-carboxylation of glutamate residues in the liver, particularly the coagulation factors VII, IX, X, prothrombin, protein C and protein S.

200. *A 25-year-old male is diagnosed as having factor VIII deficiency. The following statements are correct.*

 A. The prothrombin time is normal.
 B. Aspirin and non-steroidal anti-inflammatory drugs (NSAIDs) can safely be administered in these patients.
 C. Cryoprecipitates are preferred to factor VIII concentrates in severe disease.
 D. Desmopressin acetate is used to treat minor bleeding.
 E. ε-Aminocaproic acid can be used to control mucous bleeding.

 A.......... B.......... C.......... D.......... E..........

201. *A 40-year-old female patient is diagnosed as having DIC. The following are recognised features:*

 A. low platelet count.
 B. low serum fibrinogen levels.
 C. low fibrinogen degradation products (FDPs).
 D. prolonged thrombin time.
 E. microangiopathic haemolysis.

 A.......... B.......... C.......... D.......... E..........

202. *Heparin*

 A. potentiates the effects of antithrombin III.
 B. causes thrombocytopenia.
 C. anticoagulation is reversed instantly on cessation of heparin infusion.
 D. is administered intramuscularly for prophylaxis.
 E. crosses the placenta.

 A.......... B.......... C.......... D.......... E..........

203. *Warfarin*

 A. has minimal effect on vitamin K-dependent coagulation factors.
 B. crosses the placenta.
 C. anticoagulation returns to normal several days after discontinuation of warfarin therapy.
 D. causes skin necrosis in protein C deficiency.
 E. therapy is monitored using the INR.

 A.......... B.......... C.......... D.......... E..........

200. A. T   B. F   C. F   D. T   E. T

The prothrombin time and bleeding time are normal in haemophilia A whereas aPTT is prolonged. Aspirin and NSAIDs should not be administered in these patients. Factor VIII concentrate is the therapy of choice in severe disease. Cryoprecipitate contains factor VIII, vWF and fibrinogen. Several bags of cryoprecipitate would be required to obtain therapeutic levels of factor VIII; hence factor VIII concentrate is used. The latter is less likely to carry a risk of viral transmission. Desmopressin acetate is used to treat minor bleeding as it increases factor VIII levels four-fold in mild or moderate haemophilia A. ε-Aminocaproic acid, an inhibitor of fibrinolysis, can be used to control mucous bleeding (e.g. following dental surgery).

201. A. T   B. T   C. F   D. T   E. T

Laboratory findings in DIC include low platelet count, low serum fibrinogen levels, increased fibrinogen degradation products (FDPs) and prolonged thrombin time and aPTT. Microangiopathic haemolysis may also occur. Causes of DIC include infections (Gram-negative septicaemia, meningococcaemia), malignant tumours, acute leukaemias (promyelocytic leukaemia), hepatic disorders, connective tissue disorders, snake and spider bites, obstetric complications (particularly abruptio placentae), shock, massive burns or trauma. The management of DIC is the treatment of the underlying condition.

202. A. T   B. T   C. F   D. F   E. T

Heparin potentiates the effects of antithrombin III resulting in immediate prolongation of thrombin time, aPTT and to a lesser extent prothrombin time. Its half-life in circulation is about 90 min and reversal of anticoagulation generally occurs within hours after cessation of heparin infusion. More rapid reversal of heparin effects may be achieved with protamine sulphate. Heparin is administered parenterally, either subcutaneously or intravenously; intramuscular injections should be minimised to avoid intramuscular haemotomas. It causes thrombocytopenia and hence periodic platelet counts should be obtained in all patients on heparin therapy. It does not cross the placenta and is used for anticoagulation in pregnancy.

203. A. F   B. T   C. T   D. T   E. T

Warfarin acts by interfering with the carboxylation of vitamin K-dependent coagulation factors. Factor VII activity declines by 6 h, factor IX by 24 h and factor X and prothrombin by 48 h. It crosses the placenta and has been implicated in fetal defects and death. Reversal of anticoagulation occurs several days after discontinuation of warfarin therapy and this may be hastened by the administration of vitamin K. Warfarin causes skin necrosis in protein C deficiency; characteristically a microvascular thrombosis occurs 3–10 days following initiation of warfarin treatment. Therapy is monitored using prothrombin time. However, as the reagents used for prothrombin time are variable, the INR is used to standardise warfarin anticoagulation. Once the warfarin dose is stable, the INR is determined approximately every fortnight.

204. *The following statements about anaemia are correct.*

   A. Circulating red cell mass actually increases.
   B. The haemoglobin is normal immediately after acute blood loss.
   C. The reticulocyte count is an indicator of bone marrow response to anaemia.
   D. Reticulocytes decrease MCV.
   E. Iron-deficiency anaemia without menstrual blood loss is usually due to gastrointestinal blood loss.

   A............   B...........   C...........   D...........   E...........

205. *The following statements about aplastic anaemia are correct.*

   A. Leucocyte count is normal.
   B. Most cases are due to drugs.
   C. Transfusion with blood products from family members should be avoided while bone marrow transplant is being considered.
   D. It is associated with myelodysplastic syndromes.
   E. Patients should be instructed to consult a physician when the temperature exceeds 38.5°C.

   A............   B...........   C...........   D...........   E...........

206. *Recognised features of iron-deficiency anaemia include*

   A. pica.
   B. koilonychia.
   C. pencil cells in blood smear.
   D. raised serum ferritin level.
   E. therapeutic response to blood transfusion is superior to iron replacement.

   A............   B...........   C...........   D...........   E...........

204.   A. F   B. T   C. T   D. F   E. T

Anaemia is defined as a decrease in circulating red cell mass and the usual indices of measurement include haemoglobin and haematocrit. The haemoglobin is normal immediately after acute blood loss because compensatory mechanisms have not yet restored the plasma volume. The reticulocyte count is an indicator of bone marrow response to anaemia as it reflects red cell production. Reticulocytes are larger than mature red blood cells and will raise the MCV. Iron-deficiency anaemia without menstrual blood loss is usually due to gastrointestinal blood loss.

205.   A. F   B. F   C. T   D. T   E. T

Aplastic anaemia is due to absence of bone marrow stem cells and manifests with anaemia, leucopenia and thrombocytopenia. Patients should be instructed to consult a physician when the temperature exceeds 38.5°C. Fever with low neutrophil counts requires clinical examination and cultures of blood and potential sites of infection. Most cases are idiopathic, although about one-fifth are due to drugs (anticonvulsants, chloramphenicol, phenylbutazone, gold and sulphonamides) and viral disorders (hepatitis A, Epstein–Barr virus and cytomegalovirus infections). Transfusion with blood products from family members should be avoided while bone marrow transplant is being considered. Aplastic anaemia is associated with myelodysplastic syndromes, paroxysmal nocturnal haemoglobinuria and acute leukaemia.

206.   A. T   B. T   C. T   D. F   E. F

Clinical features of iron-deficiency anaemia include evidence of blood loss, a history of pica (ingestion of clay, starch or mud) and spoon-shaped nails (koilonychia). In Plummer–Vinson syndrome it is associated with difficulty in swallowing, oesophageal webs and glossitis. The MCV is decreased (microcytic picture) with pencil cells and occasional target cells. A low serum iron reflects diminished iron stores, serum iron may be low and iron-binding capacity is increased. Replacement is usually with oral ferrous sulphate and rarely with parenteral iron. Blood transfusion is not recommended for replacement of iron.

207.   *The following statements about thalassaemias are correct.*

A. In β-thalassaemia, red cell damage is due to the insoluble tetramers formed by the excess of α-globin chains.
B. The loss of all four α-globin genes causes hydrops fetalis.
C. Cooley's anaemia or thalassaemia major is due to reduced production of α-globin genes.
D. Red blood cell transfusions prevent skeletal deformities.
E. Large doses of vitamin C should be administered during iron chelation therapy. (F)

A............   B..........   C..........   D..........   E..........

208.   *Causes of sideroblastic anaemia include*

A. lead toxicity.
B. pyridoxine therapy.
C. ethanol.
D. isoniazid therapy.
E. malignancy.

A............   B..........   C..........   D..........   E..........

209.   *Causes of folic acid deficiency include*

A. chronic blood loss.
B. alcoholism.
C. haemolytic anaemia.
D. pregnancy.
E. anticonvulsant therapy.

A............   B..........   C..........   D..........   E..........

207.   A. T   B. T   C. F   D. T   E. F

The thalassaemias are due to underproduction of either α- or β-globin chains of the haemoglobin molecule. There are four α- and two β-globin genes in normal red cells and production of the α- and β chains is equal. In β-thalassaemia, there is diminished production of β chains with normal production of α chains. In β-thalassaemia, red cell damage is due to the insoluble tetramers formed by the excess of α-globin chains; in α-thalassaemia, the tetramers formed by the β chains are more soluble, resulting in the clinical severity being milder. However, the loss of all four α-globin genes causes hydrops fetalis. Depending on the severity β-thalassaemia is categorised into three main types: thalassaemia trait, thalassaemia intermedia and Cooley's anaemia or thalassaemia major. The latter is caused by the dysfunction of both β-globin genes resulting in severe anaemia. The free α chains in β-thalassaemia form highly unstable aggregates that precipitate within the red cell precursors in the form of insoluble inclusions. A number of untoward effects follow, the most important being damage to the cell membrane leading to loss of potassium and impaired DNA synthesis. The net effect is destruction of red cell precursors in the bone marrow, a phenomenon called ineffective erythropoiesis. The management of thalassaemia entails frequent red blood cell transfusion to improve exercise tolerance, prevent skeletal deformities and sustain life. In severe thalassaemia, massive tissue iron deposition may occur and is prevented by iron chelation therapy with desferrioxamine. Vitamin C supplementation therapy should be given with the latter, as it increases urinary iron excretion. However, large doses of vitamin C may cause release of large amounts of iron that may precipitate cardiac failure. In thalassaemia major, bone marrow transplantation should be considered in those who have HLA-identical related donors.

208.   A. T   B. F   C. T   D. T   E. T

Sideroblastic anaemia is considered to be a myelodysplastic syndrome and causes include lead toxicity, drugs including isoniazid and chloramphenicol, alcoholism, neoplasms and chronic infection. Some cases of sideroblastic anaemia may respond to pyridoxine therapy. Most patients are treated with packed red blood cells and serum erythropoietin. Bone marrow transplantation should be considered in those who have HLA-identical related donors.

209.   A. F   B. T   C. T   D. T   E. T

Causes of folic acid deficiency include alcoholism, malabsorption, haemolytic anaemia, pregnancy and drugs including anticonvulsant therapy, trimethoprim, methotrexate, sulphasalazine, pyrimethamine and oral contraceptives.

210. *Causes of vitamin B$_{12}$ deficiency include*

A. gastrectomy.
B. ileal resection.
C. *diphyllobothrium latum* infestation.
D. pancreatic insufficiency.
E. bacterial overgrowth in intestine.

A.......... B.......... C.......... D.......... E..........

211. *The following statements about megaloblastic anaemias are correct.*

A. Folic acid deficiency causes loss of vibration and positional sense.
B. Hypersegmented neutrophils are common.
C. Serum folate is a more accurate indicator of body folate stores than red blood cell folate.
D. Serum homocysteine is elevated in vitamin B$_{12}$ deficiency.
E. Empirical therapy with folic acid alone is recommended in most patients.

A.......... B.......... C.......... D.......... E..........

212. *The following statements about the anaemia of chronic renal failure are correct.*

A. Burr cells are characteristically absent.
B. Erythropoietin therapy may relieve the pruritus before the correction of anaemia.
C. Use of erythropoietin may cause iron-deficency anaemia.
D. Aluminium intoxication during haemodialysis may blunt the response to erythropoietin.
E. In secondary hyperparathyroidism, increase in erythropoietin sensitivity may occur.

A.......... B.......... C.......... D.......... E..........

210. A. T   B. T   C. T   D. T   E. T

Causes of vitamin B_{12} deficiency include intrinsic factor deficiency (pernicious anaemia, gastrectomy), ileal resection, diffuse intestinal disease (lymphoma, systemic sclerosis), *Diphyllobothrium latum* (fish tapeworm) infestation, pancreatic insufficiency and bacterial overgrowth in intestine. Other causes include pregnancy, hyperthyroidism and disseminated cancer. The feature that sets pernicious anaemia apart from other vitamin B_{12} deficiency megaloblastic anaemias is the cause of vitamin B_{12} malabsorption: atrophic gastritis with failure of production of intrinsic factor. Very little vitamin B_{12} is present in plants and vegetables and thus vegans do not obtain sufficient quantities in their diet.

211. A. F   B. T   C. F   D. F   E. F

Folic acid deficiency does not result in neurological deficits unlike vitamin B_{12} deficiency, which is associated with loss of vibrational and positional sense, paraesthesias and dementia. The blood picture in megaloblastic anaemias includes macrocytes and often thrombocytopenia and leucopenia. The neutrophils have more than five nuclear lobes (i.e. hypersegmented). Often there is ineffective erythropoiesis and premature destruction of red blood cells, resulting in elevated serum LDH and indirect bilirubin. Red cell folate is a more accurate indicator of body folate stores than serum folate. When vitamin B_{12} and folate levels are equivocal, estimation of serum homocysteine and serum methylmalonic acid are useful. Both are elevated in vitamin B_{12} deficiency, whereas serum homocysteine is elevated in folic acid deficiency. Vitamin B_{12} is required for two reactions in humans. The first is transmethylation of homocysteine to methionine, the methyl group being regenerated from folic acid. Also single-carbon formate groups derived from methionine are required for synthesis of folate polyglutamates. Thus, the lack of folate is the proximate cause of anaemia in vitamin B_{12} deficiency. In addition to the transmethylation reaction, vitamin B_{12} is required for the isomerisation of methylmalonyl coenzyme A to succinyl coenzyme A. Vitamin B_{12} deficiency thus interrupts the succinyl pathway and affects synthesis of neuronal lipids and promotes myelin breakdown causing neurological defects. Empirical therapy with folic acid alone is not recommended, as the anaemia of unrecognised vitamin B_{12} deficiency may partially respond whilst the neurological damage deteriorates further.

212. A. F   B. T   C. T   D. T   E. F

The anaemia of chronic renal failure is normochromic with occasional burr (echinocytes) and spur (acanthocytes) cells. Erythropoietin therapy may relieve the pruritus before the correction of anaemia. Use of erythropoietin may cause iron-deficiency anaemia, hypertension in one-third of the patients and seizures. Aluminium intoxication during haemodialysis may blunt the response to erythropoietin. In secondary hyperparathyroidism where there is bone marrow fibrosis, erythropoietin resistance may be seen.

213. *Recognised features of extravascular haemolysis include*

A. markedly decreased serum haptoglobin.
B. increased free haemoglobin in urine.
C. haemosiderin in the urine.
D. splenomegaly.
E. jaundice.

A........... B.......... C.......... D.......... E..........

214. *The following statements about sickle cell disease are correct.*

A. Sickle cell trait usually never occurs in those who are heterozygous for haemoglobin S.
B. Patients with sickle cell trait have an increased risk of sudden death with strenuous exercise.
C. Howell–Jolly bodies are seen in the peripheral smear.
D. Haemoglobin electrophoresis will distinguish sickle cell trait from sickle cell disease.
E. Flying in an unpressurised aircraft can precipitate sickling.

A........... B.......... C.......... D.......... E..........

215. *Recognised complications of sickle cell disease include*

A. increased incidence of premature delivery.
B. osteonecrosis of femoral heads.
C. *salmonella* osteomyelitis.
D. cholelithiasis.
E. aplastic crisis.

A........... B.......... C.......... D.......... E..........

216. *The following statements regarding hereditary spherocytosis (HS) are correct.*

A. Deficiency of spectrin is the most common abnormality in all forms of HS.
B. There is mutation in the ankyrin gene.
C. Splenectomy corrects the spherocytosis.
D. Spherocytosis is pathgnomonic of this disorder.
E. Splenectomy improves the anaemia.

A........... B.......... C.......... D.......... E..........

213. A. F   B. F   C. F   D. T   E. T

Extravascular haemolysis occurs primarily in the spleen and manifests with splenomegaly and jaundice. Haptoglobin levels are usually normal or only slightly reduced. In intravascular haemolysis haptoglobin is markedly decreased. Free haemoglobin is present in the urine in intravascular haemolysis. The presence of haemosiderin indicates chronic intravascular haemolysis, as haemosiderin can be detected in the urine usually a week after haemolysis. Intravascular haemolysis is manifested by haemoglobinaemia, haemoglobinuria, methalbuminaemia, jaundice and haemosiderinuria.

214. A. F   B. T   C. T   D. T   E. T

Sickle cell trait occurs in those who are heterozygous for haemoglobin S. Patients with sickle cell trait have an increased risk of sudden death with strenuous exercise. In sickle cell trait 40% of the haemoglobin is haemoglobin S, the rest being haemoglobin A, which interacts only weakly with haemoglobin S during the processes of gelation. Therefore, the heterozygote exhibits little tendency to sickle except under conditions of severe hypoxia. Sickling is precipitated by dehydration and hypoxia. High altitude flying, strenuous exercise and flying in an unpressurised aircraft can precipitate sickling. Blood smear shows sickle-shaped red blood cells, Howell–Jolly bodies and target cells. Haemoglobin electrophoresis will distinguish sickle cell trait from sickle cell disease. Newborns do not manifest sickle cell anaemia until 5 or 6 months of age, when the amount of fetal haemoglobin in the cells begins to reach adult levels. Fetal haemoglobin contains γ-globin chains that do not interact with haemoglobin S.

215. A. T   B. T   C. T   D. T   E. T

Complications of sickle cell disease include increased incidence of premature delivery and fetal mortality in pregnancy, osteonecrosis of femoral and humeral heads, leg ulcers, proliferative retinopathy, priapism, renal tubular damage, cholelithiasis, aplastic crisis, vaso-occlusive crisis, sequestration crisis and osteomyelitis due to *Salmonella* and *Staphylococcus* in adults and *Streptococcus pneumoniae* and *Haemophilus influenzae* in children.

216. A. T   B. T   C. F   D. F   E. T

Deficiency of the red cell membrane cytoskeletal protein spectrin is the most common abnormality in all forms of HS. Mutation of the ankyrin (another membrane cytoskeletal protein) gene and the consequent reduction in ankyrin synthesis results in a secondary reduction in the assembly of spectrin on the membrane. In addition, primary defects of the transmembrane transporter, protein 3 may also occur. Regardless of the primary defect, the deficiency of spectrin causes membrane instability. The loss of membrane causes the cells to assume the smallest possible diameter, namely a sphere. The important role of the spleen in the premature destruction of red cells is proved by the beneficial effect of splenectomy, following which the spherocytosis persists but the anaemia improves. Spherocytosis is not pathgnomonic of this disorder, as it is also seen in autoimmune haemolytic anaemias.

217. *The following associations are correct.*

A. Hereditary spherocytosis–positive Coombs' test.
B. Glucose 6-phosphate dehydrogenase deficiency–Heinz bodies.
C. Warm antibody autoimmune haemolytic anaemia–lymphoma.
D. Cold agglutinin disease–*Mycoplasma pneumoniae*.
E. Paroxysmal nocturnal haemoglobinuria–negative acid haemolysis test.

A.......... B.......... C.......... D.......... E..........

218. *The following statements about transfusions are correct.*

A. Leucocyte-depleting filters are required for fresh frozen plasma.
B. For immunocompromised patients, irradiation of blood products is generally recommended.
C. Cross-matching involves testing the patient's serum for antibodies against antigens on the donor's erythrocytes.
D. Platelet transfusions are usually necessary in chronic thrombocytopenia even in the absence of bleeding or coagulation defects.
E. Fresh frozen plasma transfusion is indicated to increase the level of clotting factors in patients with a documented deficiency.

A.......... B.......... C.......... D.......... E..........

219. *The following statements about the adverse reactions of transfusion are correct.*

A. Transfusion-associated graft-versus-host disease is said be due to the infusion of incompetent T lymphocytes.
B. Delayed haemolytic transfusion reactions are caused by an anamnestic response.
C. Over half of patients who receive platelets on a regular basis will develop antibodies against platelet antigens.
D. Massive transfusions cause hypocalcaemia.
E. Platelet transfusions are usually effective in post-transfusion purpura.

A.......... B.......... C.......... D.......... E..........

217.   A. F   B. T   C. T   D. T   E. F

In hereditary spherocytosis, the osmotic fragility test is positive and the Coombs' test is negative. In glucose 6-phosphate dehydrogenase (G6PD) deficiency, the smear shows 'bite' cells and inclusion (Heinz) bodies in the red blood cell. In G6PD-deficient cells, regeneration of reduced glutathione is impaired, causing accumulation of hydrogen peroxide. This results in the oxidation of the sulphydryl group of globin chains, which leads to denaturation of haemoglobin and formation of precipitates (Heinz bodies) within the cells. As the inclusion-bearing red cells pass through the splenic cords, macrophages pluck out the Heinz bodies giving rise to red cells that appear to have a 'bite' of cytoplasm removed. Warm antibody autoimmune haemolytic anaemia is usually caused by an anti-IgG antibody and is associated with lymphoma, chronic lymphocytic anaemia, collagen disorders and drugs. Cold agglutinin disease when chronic is associated with lymphomas and when acute with infections including *M. pneumoniae* and infectious mononucleosis. Paroxysmal nocturnal haemolytic haemoglobinuria is a disorder of bone marrow stem cells characterised by episodic intravascular haemolysis and venous thromboembolism. Ham test or positive acid haemolysis test is used to make the diagnosis. Absence of decay-accelerating factor in haemopoietic cells is also diagnostic.

218.   A. F   B. T   C. T   D. F   E. T

Patients receiving repeated and chronic transfusions are administered blood through a leucocyte-depleting filter to decrease the risk of alloimmunisation and non-haemolytic febrile reactions. All blood products that are not leucocyte-depleted require a 170–260 μm filter to prevent infusion of macroaggregrates, fibrin and debris. Leucocyte-depleting filters are not needed for fresh frozen plasma. For immunocompromised patients, irradiation of blood products is generally recommended. Cross-matching involves testing the patient's serum for antibodies against antigens on the donor's erythrocytes. Platelet transfusions are usually not necessary in chronic thrombocytopenia even in the absence of bleeding or coagulation defects. Fresh frozen plasma transfusion is used to increase the level of clotting factors in patients with deficiency.

219.   A. T   B. T   C. T   D. T   E. F

Transfusion-associated graft-versus-host disease usually occurs in immuno-compromised individuals and is said be due to the infusion of incompetent T lymphocytes. Delayed haemolytic transfusion reactions, which occur as long as 24 h to 25 days after a transfusion, are caused by an anamnestic response or a primary antibody response to erythrocyte antigens. Over half of patients who receive platelets on a regular basis will develop antibodies against platelet antigens. Massive transfusions cause hypocalcaemia by citrate intoxication. Rarely patients require intravenous calcium therapy. Calcium should never be added directly to the transfusion bottle as it can cause the blood to clot. Platelet transfusions are ineffective in post-transfusion purpura.

220. *The following statements about breast cancer are correct.*

    A. A breast lump in a postmenopausal woman is less likely to be cancerous than a breast lump in a premenopausal woman.

    B. Lumpectomy and axillary node resection is as effective as a modified radical mastectomy.

    C. The presence or absence of metastases in axillary lymph nodes is the most important prognostic factor.

    D. Oestrogen receptor-negative breast cancer that has metastasised should be treated with hormonal manipulation.

    E. Adjuvant chemotherapy has no role in the treatment of breast cancers.

    A.......... B.......... C.......... D.......... E..........

221. *The following statements about gastrointestinal malignancies are correct.*

    A. Squamous cell carcinomas of the oesophagus usually arise from Barrett's oesophagus.

    B. Adjuvant chemotherapy is usually effective in adenocarcinomas of the stomach.

    C. Colon and rectal adenocarcinomas are primarily treated by surgical resection.

    D. 5-Fluorouracil should be avoided in metastatic rectal and colon carcinomas.

    E. Anal cancers are primarily treated by surgical resection.

    A.......... B.......... C.......... D.......... E..........

222. *The following statements about genitourinary malignancies are correct.*

    A. BCG (bacille Calmette–Guérin) vaccination is used in the treatment of multifocal transitional cell carcinoma of the bladder.

    B. Cigarette smoking has been implicated in the causation of transitional cell carcinoma of the bladder.

    C. Prostate-specific antigen is a useful marker of prostatic carcinoma.

    D. Chemotherapy is the mainstay in the management of prostatic carcinoma.

    E. Cancer of the testis is usually resistant to chemotherapy.

    A.......... B.......... C.......... D.......... E..........

223. *The following statements are correct.*

    A. Ovarian cancer is primarily a disease of premenopausal women.

    B. The serum marker CA-125 is elevated in the majority of patients with epithelial ovarian cancer.

    C. Despite aggressive surgical and radiation therapy, approximately two-thirds of patients with head and neck cancer have uncontrolled local disease.

    D. Abdominal hysterectomy should be avoided in microinvasive cervical cancers.

    E. Metastatic cervical cancers are treated with cisplatin-based chemotherapy.

    A.......... B.......... C.......... D.......... E..........

220. A. F   B. T   C. T   D. F   E. F

A breast lump in a postmenopausal woman is more likely to be cancerous than a breast lump in a premenopausal woman. In premenopausal women the breast lump should be observed for 1 month to identify cyclic changes. Bilateral mammography must be performed when a lump is found in one breast. Lumpectomy and axillary node resection is as effective as a modified radical mastectomy. Axillary lymph node dissection should be included as the presence or absence of metastases in axillary lymph nodes is the most important prognostic factor. Oestrogen receptor-negative breast cancer that has metastasised usually does not respond to hormonal manipulation. Adjuvant chemotherapy should be administered to premenopausal women with axillary lymph node involvement. In postmenopausal individuals, adjuvant chemotherapy may be of benefit in oestrogen receptor-negative tumours whereas oestrogen receptor-positive patients should be treated with tamoxifen.

221. A. F   B. F   C. T   D. F   E. F

Adenocarcinomas usually arise from Barrett's oesophagus. Adjuvant chemotherapy is usually ineffective in gastric adenocarcinomas. Surgical therapy is curative in localised gastric adenocarcinomas. Colon and rectal adenocarcinomas are primarily treated by surgical resection. 5-Fluorouracil is the mainstay of treatment for metastatic colon or rectal cancer. Anal cancers treated with chemotherapy and radiation have a higher cure rate than surgery and allows the sphincter to remain intact. Surgery in anal cancers is used only as salvage therapy.

222. A. T   B. T   C. T   D. F   E. F

BCG vaccination and mitomycin C are used in the treatment of multifocal transitional cell carcinoma of the bladder. Cigarette smoking has been implicated in the causation of transitional cell carcinoma of the bladder. Prostate-specific antigen is a useful marker of prostatic carcinoma, particularly to determine recurrence, bulk of disease and response to therapy. The role of chemotherapy in prostatic carcinoma has not yet been established. Cancer of the testis is one of the most curable tumours when treated with chemotherapy. Most patients with seminoma, however, should be treated with radiation therapy.

223. A. F   B. T   C. T   D. F   E. T

Ovarian cancer is primarily a disease of postmenopausal women. The serum marker CA-125 is elevated in the majority of patients with epithelial ovarian cancer. Despite aggressive surgical and radiation therapy, approximately two-thirds of patients with head and neck cancer have uncontrolled local disease. Risk factors for cervical cancer include multiple sexual partners, multiparity and human papilloma virus. Abdominal hysterectomy should be performed in microinvasive cervical cancers. Metastatic cervical cancers are treated with cisplatin-based chemotherapy.

224. *The following statements about lung cancer are correct.*

A. In non-small-cell lung cancer, surgical resection affords the best chance of cure.
B. In patients with small-cell lung cancer who achieve complete remission with chemotherapy, prophylactic whole-brain radiation therapy may be administered to decrease the risk of CNS relapse.
C. Adjuvant chemotherapy improves survival in non-small-cell lung cancer after surgical resection.
D. In patients with metastatic non-small-cell lung cancer, cisplatin-based combination chemotherapy may modestly improve survival.
E. Paraneoplastic syndromes are more commonly associated with non-small-cell tumours than with small-cell cancer.

A.......... B.......... C.......... D.......... E..........

225. *The following statements about malignant melanoma are correct.*

A. The depth of invasion is inversely related to the prognosis.
B. Adjuvant radiotherapy improves the results of surgery.
C. Enlarging naevi that are suspicious of melanoma should be removed by excisional biopsy.
D. Metastatic systemic disease may respond to chemotherapy.
E. Malignant melanoma should be suspected when there is a change in the colour in a pigmented lesion.

A.......... B.......... C.......... D.......... E..........

226. *The following statements about sarcomas are correct.*

A. They arise from mesenchymal tissue.
B. They rarely occur in bone.
C. Haematogenous spread to the lungs is rare.
D. The prognosis of soft-tissue sarcoma is primarily determined by the cell of origin.
E. Surgical resection with adjuvant chemotherapy is used in the management of osteogenic sarcomas.

A.......... B.......... C.......... D.......... E..........

227. *The following statements about malignancies arising from unknown primary sites are correct.*

A. Usually, systemic therapy is beneficial if the primary site is identified.
B. Chemotherapy does not improve survival compared to palliative therapy.
C. When squamous cell carcinoma is identified in cervical lymph nodes the patient is presumed to have primary head and neck cancer.
D. Midline mass in the mediastinum should be investigated for extragonadal germ cell tumours.
E. Radiation therapy may be curative in squamous cell carcinomas of the head and neck.

A.......... B.......... C.......... D.......... E..........

224. A. T   B. T   C. F   D. T   E. F

In non-small-cell lung cancer, surgical resection affords the best chance of cure. In patients with small-cell lung cancer who achieve complete remission with chemotherapy, prophylactic whole-brain radiation therapy may be administered to decrease the risk of CNS relapse. Adjuvant chemotherapy or radiotherapy do not improve survival in non-small-cell lung cancer after surgical resection. In patients with metastatic non-small-cell lung cancer, cisplatin-based combination chemotherapy may modestly improve survival. Paraneoplastic syndromes are more commonly associated with small-cell tumours than with non-small-cell cancer.

225. A. T   B. F   C. T   D. T   E. T

The depth of invasion is inversely related to the prognosis. Adjuvant radiotherapy or chemotherapy does not improve the results of surgery. Enlarging naevi that suggest melanoma should be removed by exicisional biopsy. Metastatic systemic disease may respond to dacarbazine, interferon-α or interleukin-2 in about one-fifth of patients. The most important clinical sign of the disease is change in colour in a pigmented lesion.

226. A. T   B. F   C. F   D. F   E. T

Sarcomas arise from mesenchymal tissue. They commonly occur in bone or soft tissue. Haematogenous spread to the lungs is common and all patients should have a CT scan of the chest. The prognosis of soft-tissue sarcoma is primarily determined by the tumour grade and not by the cell of origin. Surgical resection with adjuvant chemotherapy is used in the management of osteogenic sarcomas.

227. A. T   B. T   C. T   D. T   E. T

Metastatic disease arising from unidentifiable primary sites is found in many patients, despite clinical examination, routine laboratory investigations and chest X-ray. The search for the primary site depends on the histopathology and the site of metastasis. Specific tissue antigens, using immunohistochemical stains, help to define the origin of the tumour. Usually, systemic therapy is beneficial if the primary site is identified. Chemotherapy does not improve survival compared with palliative therapy. Squamous cell carcinoma in cervical lymph nodes is usually presumed to be from primary head and neck cancer. Radiation therapy may be curative in squamous cell carcinomas of the head and neck. Midline mass in the mediastinum should be investigated for extragonadal germ cell tumours, initially measuring α-fetoprotein and β-human chorionic gonadotrophin levels in serum. Extragonadal germ cell tumours are potentially curable.

228. *The following statements about Hodgkin's lymphoma are correct.*

A. The presence of fever and night sweats indicates a good prognosis.
B. With liver involvement patients should receive combination chemotherapy.
C. With single lymph-node enlargement and presence of drenching night sweats, chemotherapy is the treatment of choice.
D. When more than one group of lymph nodes is involved on the same side of the diaphragm and the patient has no symptoms, radiation therapy is usually the treatment of choice.
E. The cervical lymph nodes are usually involved.

A.......... B.......... C.......... D.......... E..........

229. *The following statements about leukaemias are correct.*

A. Acute non-lymphocytic leukaemia is the commonest acute leukaemia in adults.
B. Cytosine arabinoside is the cornerstone of induction therapy in acute non-lymphocytic leukaemia.
C. Chronic lymphocytic leukaemia often evolves to acute leukaemia.
D. Richter's syndrome is where chronic lymphocytic leukaemia evolves to a high-grade lymphoma.
E. Patients with uncomplicated chronic lymphocytic leukaemia without symptoms are followed-up without therapy.

A.......... B.......... C.......... D.......... E..........

230. *Recognised features of hairy cell leukaemia include the following:*

A. it is rare in males.
B. lymphadenopathy is common.
C. pancytopenia.
D. presence of tartrate-resistant acid phosphatase in the affected cells.
E. it is a T-cell leukaemia.

A.......... B.......... C.......... D.......... E..........

231. *Recognised causes of gingival hypertrophy include*

A. phenytoin.
B. cyclosporin.
C. myelomonocytic leukaemia.
D. nifedipine.
E. thyrotoxicosis.

A.......... B.......... C.......... D.......... E..........

228.   A. F   B. T   C. T   D. T   E. T

Hodgkin's lymphoma usually presents with cervical lymph node involvement. Patients are staged as follows: stage I, the disease is localised to a single lymph node or group; stage II, more than one group of lymph nodes is involved but confined to the same side of the diaphragm; stage III, the disease involves the lymph nodes or spleen on both sides of the diaphragm; stage IV, there is liver or bone marrow involvement. These stages are subdivided into groups A and B. The absence of symptoms is classified as A. Symptoms of the B group include fever above 38.5°C, night sweats requiring a change of clothes and more than 10% weight loss over 6 months. The presence of these symptoms suggests that the disease is bulky and the prognosis is worse. Stages IA and IIA are treated with radiotherapy unless the mediastinal lymph node enlargement exceeds one-third of the chest. Stage IIIA is treated with either chemotherapy or radiation therapy. Stage IV or B-group symptoms regardless of stage are treated with chemotherapy.

229.   A. T   B. T   C. F   D. T   E. T

Acute non-lymphocytic leukaemia is the commonest acute leukaemia in adults. Cytosine arabinoside is the cornerstone of induction therapy in acute non-lymphocytic leukaemia. Chronic lymphocytic leukaemia does not evolve to acute leukaemia. Richter's syndrome is where chronic lymphocytic leukaemia evolves to a high-grade lymphoma. The presence of lymphocytosis alone without symptoms is not an indication for therapy in chronic lymphocytic leukaemia.

230.   A. F   B. F   C. T   D. T   E. F

Hairy cell leukaemia is a chronic B-cell disorder with the characteristic tartrate-resistant acid phosphatase in the affected cells. It occurs in older males and its manifestations result largely from infiltration of the liver, spleen and bone marrow. Lymphadenopathy is rare and pancytopenia occurs in more than half the cases.

231.   A. T   B. T   C. T   D. T   E. F

Gingival hypertrophy occurs in therapy with phenytoin, cyclosporin and nifedipine. It is also associated with myelomonocytic leukaemia.

6 INFECTIOUS DISEASES

232. *The following statements are correct.*

   A. Live vaccines are more likely to induce long-term immunity compared with killed vaccines.
   B. Most killed vaccines induce active immunity in the majority of recipients after a single dose.
   C. Intramuscular hepatitis B vaccine gives a diminished immune response when injected in the buttocks compared with the deltoids.
   D. Measles, mumps and rubella vaccine can be administered with the oral polio vaccine.
   E. Immune globulin may interfere with the take of live measles vaccine.

   A.......... B.......... C.......... D.......... E..........

233. *The following statements are correct.*

   A. Pneumococcal vaccine should be avoided in patients with known HIV infection.
   B. Oral polio vaccine can be safely administered to pregnant women.
   C. Tetanus toxoid can be safely administered to pregnant women.
   D. Rubella vaccine is contraindicated in women of child-bearing age.
   E. Mumps vaccine is best avoided in young males.

   A.......... B.......... C.......... D.......... E..........

234. *The following statements about hepatitis B vaccine are correct.*

   A. It can prevent hepatitis B-related liver cancer.
   B. It is derived from inserting the gene for HBsAg into *Saccharomyces cerevisiae*.
   C. Universal infant vaccination is now recommended.
   D. It is administered intravenously.
   E. The duration of vaccine-conferred immunity is not known.

   A.......... B.......... C.......... D.......... E..........

232. A. T   B. F   C. T   D. T   E. T

Live vaccines usually induce immune responses more closely resembling natural infection and thus are more likely to induce long-term immunity and are usually effective in inducing active immunity in the majority of recipients after a single dose. Killed vaccines (inactivated vaccines or toxoids), which contain large quantities of antigen, require multiple doses.

233. A. F   B. F   C. T   D. F   E. F

Patients with HIV infection should receive pneumococcal vaccine and annual influenza vaccine. In general, live vaccines should be avoided in pregnant women because of theoretical risks to the fetus; polio and yellow fever vaccines should not be given to pregnant women unless there is a substantial risk of disease. Tetanus toxoid is particularly indicated in pregnant women who are not vaccinated to protect the fetus from neonatal tetanus. Rubella vaccine is especially indicated for susceptible females of child-bearing age; mumps vaccine is indicated for patients who do not have active immunity to mumps, especially susceptible males.

234. A. T   B. T   C. T   D. F   E. T

Hepatitis B vaccine is the first vaccine that can prevent liver cancer, in addition to preventing the acute and chronic complications of hepatitis B. Currently produced vaccines are derived from inserting the gene for HBsAg into *Saccharomyces cerevisiae*. The duration of immunity conferred is not known, although it has been documented that it confers immunity within 11 years of vaccination; however, booster doses are not currently recommended. It is given intramuscularly and the major side-effect is soreness at the injection site.

235. *β-Lactam antimicrobials*

  A. exclude penicillins.
  B. interefere with bacterial cell wall physiology.
  C. include cephalosporins.
  D. include carbapenems.
  E. resistance may result from alterations in the pencillin-binding proteins on the bacterial cytoplasmic membrane.

  A...........   B...........   C...........   D...........   E...........

236. *The following statements are correct.*

  A. Benzylpencillin is active against many anaerobes.
  B. Benzylpencillin is usually administered orally.
  C. Cephalosporins are drugs of first choice against enterococcal infections.
  D. Both first- and second-generation cephalosporins are drugs of choice for Gram-negative bacillary meningitis.
  E. Aztreonam is particularly effective against anerobes.

  A...........   B...........   C...........   D...........   E...........

237. *The following associations between antimicrobial agents and toxicity are correct.*

  A. Erythromycin–prolongation of QT interval.
  B. Vancomycin–red man syndrome.
  C. Tetracyclines–vaginal candidiasis.
  D. Chloramphenicol–aplastic anaemia.
  E. Aminoglycosides–ototoxicity.

  A...........   B...........   C...........   D...........   E...........

238. *The following associations between antimicrobial agents and toxicity are correct.*

  A. Sulphonamides–Stevens–Johnson syndrome.
  B. Trimethoprim–megaloblastic anemia.
  C. Metronidazole–disulfiram-like reaction with alcohol.
  D. Methicillin–interstitial nephritis.
  E. Clindamycin–pseudomembranous colitis.

  A...........   B...........   C...........   D...........   E...........

235. A. F   B. T   C. T   D. T   E. T

β-Lactam antimicrobials include pencillins, cephalosporins, carbapenems, cephamycins and monobactams. They act by binding to penicillin-binding proteins on the bacterial cytoplasmic membrane and interefere with cell wall physiology. β-Lactam resistance may result from alterations in penicillin-binding proteins on the bacterial cytoplasmic membrane, decreased permeation of the membrane by the drug or degradation of the drug by β-lactamases.

236. A. T   B. F   C. F   D. F   E. F

Benzylpencillin or penicillin G is active against many anaerobes, most Gram-positive and Gram-negative aerobic cocci. It is hydrolysed by gastric acid and is administered intramuscularly. Cephalosporin resistance is particularly common with enterococci (Enterobacter, Pseudomonas, Citrobacter) and hence cephalosporins are not indicated for the treatment of enterococcal infection. Both first- and seccond-generation cephalosporins do not cross the meninges and should not be used to treat meningitis. The third-generation cephalosporins are drugs of first choice for Gram-negative bacillary meningitis. Aztreonam, a monobactam, is inactive against anaerobes and Gram-positive cocci. It is useful in patients who are allergic to penicillin.

237. A. T   B. T   C. T   D. T   E. T

Erythromycin can prolong the QT interval and increase susceptibility to life-threatening ventricular arrhythmias. Therefore it should not be administered concurrently with H_1-receptor blockers, e.g. terfenadine or astemizole. Vancomycin can cause tingling and flushing of the face, neck and torso (the red man syndrome) and hypotension, all mediated by the release of histamine. Tetracyclines can cause oral or vaginal thrush, elevate blood urea nitrogen and adversely affect developing teeth and bones; doxycycline can cause photosensitivity. Chloramphenicol can cause an idiosyncratic but fatal aplastic anaemia in 1 in 25 000 cases. Aminoglycosides can cause ototoxicity by affecting either the cochlea or vestibule, particularly during prolonged use in patients with renal failure treated with loop diuretics. It is recommended that serial audiometry should be conducted on patients treated for extended periods.

238. A. T   B. T   C. T   D. T   E. T

Both erythema multiforme and Stevens–Johnson syndrome may occur with sulphonamides. In addition they can induce haemolytic anaemia in patients with G6PD deficiency, crystalluria and hypersensitivity reaction (includes skin rashes, fever, vasculitis). Trimethoprim can induce megaloblastic anaemia and bone marrow suppression as a result of the inhibiton of folate metabolism. Metronidazole toxicity includes alterations in taste such as metallic taste, disulfiram-like effects with alcohol, neuropathy and teratogenicity. Clindamycin causes diarrhoea, rash and pseudomembranous colitis.

239.   *The following statements about the antimicrobial spectrum of antibiotics are correct.*

A. Ciprofloxacin is ineffective against *Pseudomonas aeruginosa*.
B. Metronidazole is also active against parasites.
C. Isoniazid is bacteriostatic against *Mycobacterium tuberculosis*.
D. Pyrazinamide is bactericidal for intracellular mycobacteria.
E. Rifampicin is bactericidal for most species of *Mycobacterium*.

A............   B..........   C..........   D..........   E..........

240.   *The following statements about antiviral drugs are correct.*

A. Amantadine is effective against infections caused by influenza B virus.
B. Acyclovir is used to treat varicella-zoster virus infections.
C. Ganciclovir is more active than acyclovir against cytomegalovirus.
D. Foscarnet has antiviral activity against herpes viruses and HIV.
E. Zidovudine is a retroviral agent used for therapy of HIV disease.

A............   B..........   C..........   D..........   E..........

241.   *The following statements about antifungal agents are correct.*

A. Amphotericin B is indicated for most systemic mycoses.
B. Flucytosine is used in combination with amphotericin B in the treatment of cryptococcal meningitis.
C. Ketoconazole penetrates readily into the cerebrospinal fluid (CSF).
D. Itraconazole has a broad antifungal spectrum.
E. Miconazole is the drug of choice in *Pseudallescheria* infection.

A............   B..........   C..........   D..........   E..........

242.   *The following statements about bacterial septicaemia are correct.*

A. A first-generation cephalosporin plus an aminoglycoside will cover most potential pathogens of community-acquired septicaemia.
B. Post-splenectomy patients are particularly susceptible to septicaemia due to encapsulated organisms.
C. Vancomycin plus an aminoglycoside is appropriate therapy for sepsis due to nosocomial pathogens.
D. Corticosteroids at high doses significantly improve the ultimate outcome in septic shock.
E. In early bacteraemic shock, cardiac output may be elevated.

A............   B..........   C..........   D..........   E..........

239. A. F   B. T   C. F   D. T   E. T

Ciprofloxacin like other fluoroquinolones is effective against most Gram-negative bacilli including *P. aeruginosa*. Metronidazole is effective against most Gram-negative anaerobic bacteria (*Bacteroides* and *Clostridium*), protozoa and parasites (*Entamoeba histolytica, Trichomonas vaginalis, Giardia lamblia* and *Dracunculus medinensis*). Isoniazid is bactericidal for *M. tuberculosis, M. Kansasii* and *M. bovis*. Pyrazinamide is bactericidal for intracellular mycobacteria and rifampicin is bactericidal for most species of *Mycobacterium*, Gram-positive cocci and many Gram-negative bacilli.

240. A. F   B. T   C. T   D. T   E. T

Amantadine blocks an early step in the replication of the influenza A virus and has no effect on infections caused by influenza B or C. Acyclovir is active against herpes simplex virus (types 1 and 2) and the varicella–zoster virus. Its clinical utility against cytomegalovirus and Epstein–Barr virus is under question. Ganciclovir is more active than acyclovir against cytomegalovirus and Epstein–Barr virus. Foscarnet has antiviral activity against herpes viruses and HIV. Zidovudine is a retroviral agent used for therapy of HIV disease.

241. A. T   B. T   C. F   D. T   E. T

Amphotericin B is indicated for most systemic mycoses except *Pseudallescheria boydii* infections. Flucytosine is used in combination with amphotericin B in the treatment of cryptococcal meningitis. Ketoconazole penetrates cerebrospinal fluid unreliably. Fluconazole penetrates readily into the CSF and is used as maintenance therapy for cryptococcal meningitis in patients with AIDS. Itraconazole has a broad antifungal spectrum including histoplasmosis and blastomycosis in immunocompromised hosts. Miconazole is the drug of choice in *Pseudallescheria* infection.

242. A. T   B. T   C. T   D. F   E. T

A first-generation cephalosporin plus an aminoglycoside will cover most potential pathogens of community-acquired septicaemia. Post-splenectomy patients are particularly susceptible to septicaemia due to encapsulated organisms (*Neisseria meningitidis, H. influenzae, strep. pneumoniae*). Vancomycin plus an aminoglycoside is appropriate therapy for sepsis due to nosocomial pathogens (*Staphylococcus aureus*, enterococci and Gram-negative bacilli). Corticosteroids even at high doses do not significantly improve the ultimate outcome in septic shock. In early bacteraemic shock, cardiac output may be elevated.

243. *The following statements about syphilis are correct.*

A. All patients diagnosed as having syphilis should be tested for HIV infection.
B. The fluorescent treponemal antibody (FTA) test is used to monitor therapy.
C. The veneral disease research laboratory (VDRL) can be positive in systemic lupus erythematosus.
D. A single dose of 2.4 million units of benzathine pencillin is recommended for the treatment of primary syphilis.
E. Diagnosis of primary syphilis is made by dark-field microscopy.

A........... B.......... C.......... D.......... E..........

244. *Gonorrhoea*

A. in men presents as purulent urethritis.
B. is caused by diplococci.
C. specimens should be plated immediately on warm chocolate agar.
D. causes salpingitis.
E. can cause endocarditis in disseminated infection.

A........... B.......... C.......... D.......... E..........

245. *Causes of non-gonococcal urethritis include*

A. herpes simplex.
B. *Haemophilus ducreyi.*
C. *Chlamydia trachomatis.*
D. *Ureaplasma urealyticum.*
E. *T. vaginalis.*

A........... B.......... C.......... D.......... E..........

246. *The following statements about Mycobacterium infections are correct.*

A. Pyrazinamide is ineffective against *M. kansasii.*
B. *M. avium* complex characteristically spares the lymph nodes.
C. Streptomycin should be avoided in pregnant women.
D. *M. marinum* infection spares cutaneous tissues.
E. A positive tuberculin test in immigrants from Asia does not require prophylactic treatment with isoniazid.

A........... B.......... C.......... D.......... E..........

243.   A. T   B. F   C. T   D. T   E. T

All patients diagnosed as having syphilis should be tested for HIV infection. The FTA test is not used to monitor therapy as it remains positive for life. The VDRL can be positive in systemic lupus erythematosus, infectious mononucleosis, *Mycoplasma* infection and intravenous drug abusers. A single dose of 2.4 million units of benzathine pencillin is recommended for the treatment of primary syphilis. Diagnosis of primary syphilis is made by dark-field microscopy.

244.   A. T   B. T   C. T   D. T   E. T

Gonorrhoea in men presents as purulent urethritis and in women as cervicitis. *Neisseria gonorrhoeae* is a Gram-negative intracellular diplococci and is diagnostic in men, whereas in women it can be mistaken for saprophytic *Neisseria*. Diagnosis can be made by culture, for which the specimens must be plated immediately on warm chocolate agar or Thayer–Martin medium. Gonorrhoeal salpingitis is indistinguishable from that caused by other organisms. Endocarditis and meningitis may occur in patients with disseminated infection.

245.   A. F   B. F   C. T   D. T   E. T

Non-gonococcal urethritis is caused by *Chl. trachomatis* in about 40% of cases, *U. urealyticum* in another 40% and *T. vaginalis* in 5%. *Chl. trachomatis* also causes lymphogranuloma venereum. Chancroid is due to *H. ducreyi*.

246.   A. T   B. F   C. T   D. F   E. F

Pyrazinamide is ineffective against *M. kansasii*. *M. avium* complex is the most common non-tuberculous mycobacterium that causes lymphadenitis. Streptomycin and pyrazinamide should be avoided in pregnant women; isoniazid, rifampicin and ethambutol are used to treat tuberculosis in pregnant women. *M. marinum* infection affects cutaneous tissues and limited disease is treated with ciprofloxacin or doxycycline. A positive tuberculin test in immigrants from Asia requires prophylactic treatment with isoniazid.

247. *The following statements about the management of malaria are correct.*

A. Mefloquine is used as prophylaxis for travellers to areas of the world were chloroquine-resistant *Plasmodium falciparum* is present.
B. Chloroquine-resistant *P. falciparum* malaria should be treated with two drugs: quinine sulphate and doxycycline/pyrimethamine.
C. *P. vivax* infections may relapse several months after initial illness.
D. Normal G6PD levels should be documented prior to the administration of primaquine.
E. Cerebral malaria should be treated with intravenous quinidine.

A.......... B.......... C.......... D.......... E..........

248. *The following statements about HIV infection are correct.*

A. It spares cells that bear the CD4 surface marker.
B. The CD4 lymphocyte count is markedly elevated.
C. Zidovudine therapy improves survival in asymptomatic patients with normal CD4 counts.
D. Dideoxyinosine is used in the treatment if the patient has a previous history of pancreatic disease.
E. Prophylaxis against tuberculosis in patients with a positive Mantoux test is contraindicated in seropositive patients.

A.......... B.......... C.......... D.......... E..........

249. *The following associations in HIV-positive patients are correct.*

A. JC virus–progressive multifocal leucoencephalopathy.
B. Cytomegalovirus–oesophagitis.
C. *Cryptococcus neoformans*–meningitis.
D. Varicella-zoster–meningoencephalitis.
E. *Toxoplasma gondii*–encephalopathy.

A.......... B.......... C.......... D.......... E..........

250. *A 55-year-old patient presents with persistent but severe heart failure following myocardial infarction. On examination he has a pansystolic murmur over the precordium and fever. Haemoglobin is $10\,g\,dl^{-1}$, MCHC $30\,g\,dl^{-1}$, WBC count $13 \times 10^9/l$ and aspartate transaminase (AST/SGOT) $25\,IU\,l^{-1}$, ECG showed sinus rhythm and urine microscopy shows red blood cells. He requires the following:*

A. immediate cardiac catheterisation.
B. echocardiography.
C. blood cultures.
D. exercise tolerance test.
E. intravenous antibiotics.

A.......... B.......... C.......... D.......... E..........

247.   A. T   B. T   C. T   D. T   E. T

Mefloquine is used as prophylaxis for travellers to areas of the world where chloroquine-resistant *P. falciparum* is present. Chloroquine-resistant *P. falciparum* malaria should be treated with two drugs: quinine sulphate and doxycycline/ pyrimethamine. *P. vivax* infections may relapse several months after initial illness. Normal G6PD levels should be documented prior to the administration of primaquine. Cerebral malaria should be treated with intravenous quinidine.

248.   A. F   B. F   C. F   D. F   E. F

HIV affects all cells that bear the CD4 surface marker. A CD4 lymphocyte count less than $500/mm^3$ (normal $600-1500/mm^3$) indicates HIV infection. Zidovudine therapy does not improve survival in asymptomatic patients but does slow the progression of disease in those with CD4 cell counts between 200 and $500/mm^3$. Dideoxyinosine should not be used in the treatment if the patient has a previous history of pancreatic disease, because pancreatitis is a major side-effect. Seropositive patients with a positive Mantoux test or patients with chest X-ray findings of healed tuberculosis should receive prophylaxis against tuberculosis.

249.   A. T   B. T   C. T   D. T   E. T

Cytomegalovirus can cause systemic symptoms, oesophagitis, gastritis, enteritis, colitis, pancreatitis, cholecystitis, chorioretinitis, bone marrow suppression, necrotising inflammation of the adrenals and lower respiratory tract infection. Varicella–zoster can cause meningoencephalitis, recurrent disease and cranial neuritis. *C. neoformans* is the commonest fungal cause of CNS disease, particularly meningitis. *T. gondii* typically causes multiple CNS lesions with encephalopathy and focal deficits.

250.   A. F   B. T   C. T   D. F   E. T

This patient probably has infective endocarditis. At least six blood cultures from different sites should be taken before administration of intravenous antibiotics. *Strep. pneumoniae* responds to penicillin. Echocardiography is useful in determining the cause of pansystolic murmur, whether it is due to papillary muscle dysfunction or rupture of the interventricular septal defect.

251. *A 35-year-old male patient with AIDS presents with a 2-week history of unilateral frontal headache. On examination she is afebrile, mental status is normal and there are no lateralising neurological deficits. A CT head scan showed a 3 × 4 cm mass in the left frontal region surrounded by oedema. The mass enhances with intravenous contrast. The following management measures are appropriate:*

   A. lumbar puncture for cytology, cell count, protein, glucose and cultures.
   B. serum for *T. gondii* serology.
   C. treatment with combination of pyrimethamine and sulphadiazine.
   D. repeat CT head scan in 10 days time.
   E. Magnetic resonance imaging (MRI) of the brain to exclude multiple lesions.

   A.......... B.......... C.......... D.......... E..........

252. *Recognised clinical features of mumps include*

   A. congenital heart defects in fetuses of infected mothers.
   B. orchitis in prepubertal boys is common.
   C. pancreatitis.
   D. parotitis.
   E. aseptic meningitis.

   A.......... B.......... C.......... D.......... E..........

253. *Epstein–Barr virus has been implicated as a causative agent in*

   A. hairy leucoplakia in the mouth.
   B. hairy-cell leukaemia.
   C. Burkitt's lymphoma.
   D. nasopharyngeal carcinoma.
   E. lymphoproliferative disorders in transplant patients.

   A.......... B.......... C.......... D.......... E..........

254. *The following statements about* Sarcoptes scabiei *infestation are correct.*

   A. The male mites burrow into the skin.
   B. Person-to-person transmission is rare.
   C. Most normal hosts have a large number of adult organisms.
   D. The organism reproduces and matures on the human host.
   E. The organism is difficult to isolate.

   A.......... B.......... C.......... D.......... E..........

255. *Recognised clinical features of infectious mononucleosis include*

   A. splenomegaly.
   B. rash associated with ampicillin.
   C. prolonged asthenia following infection.
   D. aplastic anaemia.
   E. elevated liver enzymes.

   A.......... B.......... C.......... D.......... E..........

251.   A. F   B. T   C. T   D. T   E. T

Intracerebral mass lesions in AIDS patients are usually due to toxoplasmosis or lymphoma and lumbar punctures are not useful to confirm these diagnoses. Lumbar puncture should be avoided in such patients. Empirical therapy with pyrimethamine and sulphadiazine should begin without delay after serum samples for *Toxoplasma* serology have been taken. MRI brain scan may detect multiple lesions not seen on CT scan. Response to therapy can be assessed by serial CT head scans.

252.   A. F   B. F   C. T   D. T   E. T

There is no strong association between mumps and congenital heart defects in fetuses of infected mothers. Orchitis is more common in postpubertal males. Pancreatitis, parotitis and aseptic meningitis are all recognised features of this condition.

253.   A. T   B. F   C. T   D. T   E. T

There is no evidence that Epstein–Barr virus is related to hairy-cell leukaemia but it has been implicated as a causative agent in hairy leucoplakia of the mouth, Burkitt's lymphoma, lymphoproliferative disorders in transplant patients and nasopharyngeal carcinoma.

254.   A. F   B. F   C. F   D. T   E. F

The scabies mite (*S. scabiei*) is seen in sexually active adults and family members of infected persons, confirming a person-to-person transmission. It causes a non-specific dermatitis-like picture and hence the organism has to be isolated to make a diagnosis. The female mite burrows into the skin and lays eggs; fewer than 15 adult mites are present on an infected individual. The organism reproduces and matures on the human host as there is no intermediate host.

255.   A. T   B. T   C. T   D. T   E. T

Infectious mononucleosis is caused by Epstein–Barr virus and clinical features include splenomegaly, rash associated with ampicillin therapy, prolonged asthenia following infection including myalgic encephalomyelitis, aplastic anaemia and elevated liver enzymes.

256.   *Clinical features due to* Listeria *include*

A. neonatal granulomatosis.
B. bacteraemia.
C. endocarditis.
D. conjunctivitis.
E. meningitis.

A........... B.......... C.......... D.......... E..........

257.   *A 28-year-old male doctor from India presents with a 10-day history of fever and pain in the right upper quadrant. The patient lives in the UK and visits his family in Calcutta every 2 years. He returned from a visit to India 6 weeks ago. The patient was asymptomatic in India but on his return had noticed weight loss. On examination he is febrile and there is tenderness in the right upper quadrant with the liver just palpable. Clinical examination is otherwise unremarkable. A CT scan of the abdomen shows a non-calcified mass 5 × 5 cm in the right lobe of the liver. Plain X-ray of the abdomen is normal. The possible causes of his current illness include*

A. hepatoma.
B. echinococcal cyst.
C. pyogenic liver abscess.
D. amoebic liver abscess.
E. metastases to the liver.

A........... B.......... C.......... D.......... E..........

256.   A. T   B. T   C. T   D. T   E. T

Clinical symptoms caused by *Listeria* include neonatal granulomatosis, bacteraemia, endocarditis, conjunctivitis, septic arthritis, peritonitis and meningitis. Meningitis is the commonest of these. *Listeria monocytogenes* is a Gram-positive motile rod that is a facultative intracellular parasite found in sewage, soil, mammals, fowl and humans. It is sensitive to penicillin, tetracycline and erythromycin and resistant to oxacillin.

257.   A. T   B. F   C. T   D. T   E. T

Echinococcal cyst is unlikely because hepatic cysts are usually calcified and present acutely with abdominal pain or are detected on plain X-ray of the abdomen or ultrasound done for other reasons. His symptoms can be ascribed to any of the other four causes.

7 NEUROLOGY

258. *Multiple sclerosis*

   A. is attributable to grey matter lesions that are separated in space.
   B. is caused by mycobacteria.
   C. causes spastic paraplegia.
   D. causes retrobulbar neuritis.
   E. affects men more than women.

   A............   B...........   C...........   D...........   E...........

259. *The following statements are correct.*

   A. Progressive supranuclear palsy usually presents with loss of vertical gaze.
   B. The larger the number of triplet repeats on the Huntington's disease gene, the earlier the onset of the disease.
   C. In Friedreich's ataxia, an extensor plantar reflex is present despite an absent deep tendon reflex.
   D. In amyotrophic lateral sclerosis, there is a loss of both lower motor neurones and upper motor neurones.
   E. Orthostatic hypotension is a recognised clinical feature of Shy–Drager syndrome.

   A............   B...........   C...........   D...........   E...........

260. *The following associations are correct.*

   A. Vitamin B_{12} deficiency–Korsakoff's syndrome.
   B. Fetal alcohol syndrome–microcephaly.
   C. Methanol poisoning–retinal injury.
   D. Carbon monoxide poisoning–globus pallidus necrosis.
   E. Thiamine deficiency–Wernicke's encephalopathy.

   A............   B...........   C...........   D...........   E...........

261. *Recognised manifestations of tuberous sclerosis include*

   A. shagreen patches.
   B. ash-leaf macules.
   C. subungual fibromas.
   D. angiofibromas.
   E. cardiac myomas.

   A............   B...........   C...........   D...........   E...........

258.   A. F   B. F   C. T   D. T   E. F

Multiple sclerosis is a disorder characterised by neurological deficits, separated in time, attributable to white matter lesions separated in space. Women are affected more often than men, with an overall ratio of approximately 2 : 1. Although transmissible agents have been proposed in the pathogenesis of the disorder, all attempts to identify an agent have been unsuccessful. Unilateral visual impairment due optic neuritis or retrobulbar neuritis and spastic paraplegia are some of its common manifestations.

259.   A. T   B. T   C. T   D. T   E. T

Progressive supranuclear palsy usually presents with loss of vertical gaze. The coding region of the Huntington's disease gene contains a polymorphic trinucleotide repeat, with normal chromosomes containing 11–34 copies of the $(CAG)_n$ sequences. The larger the number of triplet repeats on the Huntington's disease gene, the earlier the onset of the disease. In Friedreich's ataxia, an extensor plantar reflex is present despite an absent deep tendon reflex. In amyotrophic lateral sclerosis, there is a loss of both lower motor neurones and upper motor neurones. Orthostatic hypotension is a recognised clinical feature of Shy–Drager syndrome.

260.   A. F   B. T   C. T   D. T   E. T

Vitamin B_{12} deficiency causes subacute combined degeneration of the spinal cord. Thiamine deficiency causes Wernicke's encephalopathy and Korsakoff's syndrome (characterised by mental disturbances and confabulation). Alcohol consumption during pregnancy can cause fetal alcohol syndrome, which has the following features: growth retardation, microcephaly, facial abnormalities, cardiac septal defects, joint abnormalities and delayed development with mental impairment. Carbon monoxide-induced hypoxia causes globus pallidus necrosis and Parkinson's syndrome. In methanol poisoning, retinal injury is probably due to degeneration of retinal ganglion cells and results in blindness.

261.   A. T   B. T   C. T   D. T   E. T

Tuberous sclerosis is characterised by angiofibromas, seizures and mental retardation. Recognised manifestations include hamartomas within the CNS, renal angiomyolipomas, retinal glial hamartomas, cardiac myomas and cysts of liver, pancreas and kidneys. Cutaneous lesions include leathery thickenings in localised patches (shagreen patches), hypopigmented areas (ash-leaf patches), subungual fibromas and angiofibromas.

262. *Recognised manifestations of neurofibromatosis include*

A. neurofibromas.
B. gliomas of the optic nerve.
C. meningiomas.
D. pigmented nodules of the iris.
E. *café-au-lait* spots.

A.......... B.......... C.......... D.......... E..........

263. *The following statements about Creutzfeldt–Jakob disease are correct.*

A. It is associated with prions.
B. There is spongiform change in the grey matter.
C. Patients have rapidly progressive dementia.
D. Most patients survive for several years after diagnosis.
E. Startle myoclonus is a recognised feature.

A.......... B.......... C.......... D.......... E..........

264. *The following statements are correct.*

A. Gait ataxia is due to a lesion in the anterior lobe of cerebellum.
B. Truncal ataxia is due to a lesion in the flocculonodular lobe of the cerebellum.
C. Limb ataxia is due to a lesion in the lateral lobes of the cerebellum.
D. Upbeat nystagmus is due to a lesion in the anterior vermis of the cerebellum.
E. Vestibular nystagmus is due to a lesion in the lateral lobes of the cerebellum.

A.......... B.......... C.......... D.......... E..........

265. *Dominant hemisphere functions include*

A. drawing ability.
B. topographic ability.
C. awareness of body and space.
D. construction.
E. dressing.

A.......... B.......... C.......... D.......... E..........

266. *The following statements are correct.*

A. Loss of two-point discrimination is due to a lesion in the frontal lobe.
B. Tactile agnosia is due to a lesion in the occipital lobe.
C. Lack of awareness that the limbs are paralysed is due to a lesion in the non-dominant parietal lobe.
D. Expressive dysphasia is due to a lesion in the Broca's area.
E. Inability to recognise a familiar face is due to a lesion in the parieto-occipital lobe.

A.......... B.......... C.......... D.......... E..........

262. A. T   B. T   C. T   D. T   E. T

Recognised features of neurofibromatosis include neurofibromas, gliomas of the optic nerve, meningiomas, pigmented nodules of the iris or Lisch nodules, and *café-au-lait* spots.

263. A. T   B. T   C. T   D. F   E. T

Creutzfeldt–Jakob disease is associated with spongiform change in the grey matter. Patients have rapidly progressive dementia, often with startle myoclonus. The disease is uniformly fatal, with an average duration of 7 months, although a few patients survive for several years. Prion protein has been implicated as the transmitting agent; this is an abnormal form of a normal cellular protein that is relatively resistant to digestion by proteinase K.

264. A. T   B. T   C. T   D. T   E. F

Gait ataxia, or inability to tandem walk, is due to a lesion in the anterior lobe of the cerebellum or palaeocerebellum. Truncal ataxia, such as titubation or drunken gait, is due to a lesion in the flocculonodular or posterior lobe of the cerebellum. Limb ataxia, especially of upper limbs, and hypotonia is due to lesions of the lateral lobes or neocerebellum. Upbeat nystagmus is caused by lesions of the anterior vermis of the cerebellum, whereas downbeat nystagmus is associated with brainstem lesions, meningoencephalitis and hypomagnesaemia. Vestibular nystagmus is due to lesions in the labyrinth, vestibular nerve or vestibular nuclei.

265. A. F   B. F   C. F   D. F   E. F

Dominant hemisphere functions include right–left orientation, finger identification and calculation. Drawing ability, topographic ability, awareness of body and space, construction, facial recognition and motor persistence are non-dominant hemisphere functions.

266. A. F   B. F   C. T   D. T   E. T

Loss of two-point discrimination indicates a parietal lobe lesion. Tactile agnosia, where patients are unable to recognise objects placed in their hands despite the fact that the sensory system of the hands and fingers is intact and there is adequate motor function, is due to a lesion in the parietal lobe. Anosognosia or lack of awareness that the limbs are paralysed is due to a lesion in the non-dominant parietal lobe, whereas the inability to recognise a familiar face is due to a lesion in the parieto-occipital lobe. Expressive dysphasia is due to a lesion in Broca's area, which is located in the posterior portion of the third left frontal gyrus. It is the motor association cortex for the face, tongue, lips and palate, and contains the motor patterns necessary to produce speech.

267. *The following statements about cranial nerve palsies are correct.*

A. The presence of pain in third cranial nerve palsy discriminates between aneurysms of the posterior communicating artery and diabetes as the cause.
B. The nuclei of the sixth cranial nerve is the medulla oblongata.
C. Sixth cranial nerve palsy is a false localising sign in increased intracranial pressure.
D. The facial nerve is predominantly a sensory nerve.
E. Bell's palsy is due to tenth cranial nerve involvement.

A.......... B.......... C.......... D.......... E..........

268. *The following statements about bacterial meningitis are correct.*

A. Antimicrobial therapy should not be instituted before CT of the brain is performed.
B. *Strep. pneumoniae* and *N. meningitidis* are responsible for most cases of bacterial meningitis in adults.
C. *H. influenzae* is a rare cause of meningitis in adults.
D. *Staph. aureus* produces high mortality despite treatment.
E. *Staph. epidermidis* meningitis is usually secondary to an infected ventricular shunt.

A.......... B.......... C.......... D.......... E..........

269. *The following statements about herpes simplex encephalitis are correct.*

A. It is the most common cause of acute sporadic encephalitis.
B. CSF changes may be absent.
C. CT head scan may demonstrate localised temporal lobe oedema.
D. Brain biopsy is imperative for diagnosis.
E. Early diagnosis can be made by polymerase chain reaction for herpes simplex virus DNA in the CSF.

A.......... B.......... C.......... D.......... E..........

270. *The following statements about coma are correct.*

A. Unilateral cerebral lesions rarely cause coma unless they have sufficient mass effect to compress the brainstem or opposite hemisphere.
B. Metabolic disorders cause coma by diffuse effects on both cerebellar hemispheres.
C. The EEG is normal in most cases.
D. Lumbar puncture should be performed if midline shift is present on CT head scan.
E. If meningitis is suspected, antibiotic therapy should not be started unless a lumbar puncture is done.

A.......... B.......... C.......... D.......... E..........

267. A. F   B. F   C. T   D. F   E. F

The presence of pain in third cranial nerve palsy discriminates poorly between aneurysms of the posterior communicating artery and diabetes as the cause. The nuclei of the sixth cranial nerve is the pons and sixth cranial nerve palsy is a false localising sign in increased intracranial pressure. The long intracranial course of the sixth nerve renders it vulnerable during increased intracranial pressure. The facial nerve is predominantly a motor nerve that supplies muscles to the face. Bell's palsy is idiopathic seventh nerve palsy; however using polymerase chain reaction, herpes simplex virus has been recently implicated as a cause.

268. A. F   B. T   C. T   D. T   E. T

Antimicrobial therapy should be instituted without delay, even before radiological procedures such as CT of the brain is performed. *Strep. pneumoniae* and *N. meningitidis* are responsible for most cases of bacterial meningitis in adults. *H. influenzae* is a rare cause of meningitis in adults. *Staph. aureus* produces high mortality despite treatment. *Staph. epidermidis* meningitis is usually secondary to an infected ventricular shunt. Gram-negative bacillary meningitis is associated with trauma to the head, neonates, elderly patients and alcoholic patients. *L. monocytogenes* is an important cause of meningitis in immunocompromised adults.

269. A. T   B. T   C. T   D. F   E. T

Herpes simplex is the most common cause of acute sporadic encephalitis. CSF changes may be minimal or absent. CT head scan may demonstrate localised temporal lobe oedema, mass effect, haemorrhage and a patchy enhancement of contrast. Electroencephalogram (EEG) in herpes simplex encephalitis may show temporal lobe slow wave changes and/or periodic complexes. Brain biopsy is no longer imperative for diagnosis. Early diagnosis can be made by polymerase chain reaction for herpes simplex virus DNA in the CSF. In suspected cases, treatment with acyclovir should be instituted immediately.

270. A. T   B. F   C. F   D. F   E. F

Unilateral cerebral lesions rarely cause coma unless they have sufficient mass effect to compress the brainstem or opposite hemisphere. Metabolic disorders cause coma by diffuse effects on both cerebral hemispheres. The EEG is abnormal in most cases and a normal EEG suggests coma due to psychogenic factors. Lumbar puncture should not be performed if midline shift is present on CT head scan. If meningitis is suspected, antibiotic therapy should be started without waiting for a lumbar puncture to be done.

271. *The following associations are correct.*

    A. Small but reactive pupils–atropine.
    B. Bilateral fixed and dilated pupil–anoxic encephalopathy.
    C. Absence of all eye movements–bilateral pontine lesion.
    D. Dysconjugate gaze–brainstem lesion.
    E. Loss of vertical gaze–midbrain lesion.

    A.......... B.......... C.......... D.......... E..........

272. *The following statements are correct.*

    A. Treatment of alcohol withdrawal seizures requires long-term therapy with chronic anticonvulsant drugs.
    B. Skull fractures increase the risk of epidural haemorrhage.
    C. In Brown-Séquard syndrome, there is contralateral pain and temperature loss below the lesion and ipsilateral weakness and proprioceptive loss.
    D. In cauda equina syndrome, the sensation in the saddle area is normal.
    E. In most cases cord compression is painless.

    A.......... B.......... C.......... D.......... E..........

273. *Neurological effects of alcohol include*

    A. degeneration of the corpus callosum.
    B. central pontine myelinolysis.
    C. rhabdomyolysis.
    D. cerebellar degeneration.
    E. peroneal muscular atrophy.

    A.......... B.......... C.......... D.......... E..........

274. *The following statements are correct.*

    A. Resting tremor occurs in cerebellar disease.
    B. Intention tremor occurs in Parkinson's disease.
    C. Postural tremor is due to hyperthyroidism.
    D. Unsteadiness when standing still that is relieved while walking indicates basal ganglia involvement.
    E. Postural tremor is due to salbutamol toxicity.

    A.......... B.......... C.......... D.......... E..........

275. *The following statements about transient ischaemic attacks (TIAs) are correct.*

    A. The symptoms usually persist for more than 72 h.
    B. Amaurosis fugax indicates ischaemia of the vertebro–basilar circulation.
    C. Approximately one-third of patients will have a cerebral infarction within 5 years.
    D. Carotid endarterectomy decreases the risk of stroke and death in patients with ipsilateral high-grade carotid stenosis.
    E. Rupture of a berry aneurysm is a common cause.

    A.......... B.......... C.......... D.......... E..........

271. A. F   B. T   C. T   D. T   E. T

Small but reactive pupils are seen in narcotic poisoning, thalamic or pontine lesions and metabolic encephalopathy. Bilateral fixed and dilated pupils are seen in anoxic encephalopathy and with atropine. Absence of all eye movements indicates bilateral pontine lesion or drug-induced ophthalmoplegia (overdose of tricyclic antidepressants, sedatives, phenytoin). Dysconjugate gaze suggests a brainstem lesion. A horizontal gaze preference indicates either a unilateral pontine or frontal lobe lesion, whereas loss of vertical gaze occurs in midbrain lesions, acute hydrocephalus and central herniation.

272. A. F   B. T   C. T   D. F   E. F

Treatment of alcohol withdrawal seizures with chronic anticonvulsant drugs is usually not required. Skull fractures increase the risk of epidural haemorrhage. In Brown-Séquard syndrome (hemisection of the spinal cord), there is contralateral pain and temperature loss below the lesion and ipsilateral weakness and proprioceptive loss. In cauda equina syndrome (compression of lower lumbar and spinal roots), sensation in the saddle area is lost and there is flaccid weakness of the lower limbs, decreased deep tendon reflexes and sphincter incontinence. In most cases cord compression presents with back pain at the level of compression, difficulty with walking and cutaneous sensory loss depending on the dermatome affected.

273. A. T   B. T   C. T   D. T   E. F

Neurological effects of alcohol include Wernicke's encephalopathy, Korsakoff's psychosis, cerebellar degeneration, Marchiafava–Bignami disease (degeneration of the corpus callosum), central pontine myelinolysis, amblyopia, epilepsy, myopathy and rhabdomyolysis.

274. A. F   B. F   C. T   D. F   E. T

Tremors are involuntary movements that result from alternate contraction and relaxation of groups of muscles, producing rhythmic oscillations about a joint or a group of joints. Postural tremor is brought on when the arms are outstretched and is due to thyrotoxicosis, drugs (salbutamol, terbutaline, lithium) and alcohol. Resting tremor occurs in Parkinson's disease while intention tremor (aggravated by voluntary movements) is a feature of cerebellar disease. Unsteadiness when standing still that is relieved while walking is primary orthostatic tremor and positron emission tomography shows increased activity in the cerebellum.

275. A. F   B. F   C. T   D. T   E. F

In TIAs the symptoms by definition last less than 24 h. Amaurosis fugax or ipsilateral monocular visual loss indicates ischaemia of the carotid circulation. Approximately one-third of patients will have a cerebral infarction within 5 years. Carotid endarterectomy decreases the risk of stroke and death in patients with ipsilateral high-grade (70–99%) carotid stenosis. Rupture of a berry aneurysm is a common cause of subarachnoid haemorrhage not TIAs.

276. *The followings statements about headache are correct.*

A. Migraines are usually bilateral.
B. The aura of classic migraine is characteristically devoid of visual manifestations.
C. Cluster headaches are commoner in females.
D. Periodicity is the hallmark of cluster headaches.
E. Sumatriptan is effective in acute vascular headaches.

A.......... B.......... C.......... D.......... E..........

277. *Recognised features of dystrophia myotonica include*

A. frontal baldness.
B. ptosis.
C. cataracts.
D. wasting of the sternomastoids.
E. cardiac conduction defects.

A.......... B.......... C.......... D.......... E..........

278. *The following statements about myasthenia gravis are correct.*

A. Edrophonium often produces temporary improvement of muscle strength.
B. The electromyogram shows that the muscle action potential produces an incremental response to repetitive nerve stimulation.
C. Anticholinesterase drugs cause exacerbation of symptoms.
D. Thymectomy is effective treatment for generalised or disabling ocular myasthenia gravis.
E. Plasmapheresis is used in the treatment of acute exacerbations.

A.......... B.......... C.......... D.......... E..........

279. *The following statements are correct.*

A. Rapidly progressive ascending paralysis occurs in Guillain-Barré syndrome.
B. Rapidly progressive proximal muscle weakness occurs in polymyositis.
C. Cranial nerve palsies occurs in botulism.
D. Generalised muscle spasm occurs in tetanus.
E. CSF protein elevated without increase in cell number occurs in myasthenia gravis.

A.......... B.......... C.......... D.......... E..........

276. A. F   B. F   C. F   D. T   E. T

Migraines are usually unilateral and the aura of classic migraine consists of visual, motor and sensory manifestations. Cluster headaches are commoner in males; periodicity is the hallmark of cluster headaches. Sumatriptan is effective treatment for acute vascular headaches, although one-third of patients have a recurrence within 24 h after therapy.

277. A. T   B. T   C. T   D. T   E. T

Recognised features of dystrophia myotonica include myotonia, frontal baldness, ptosis with a smooth forehead, cataracts, expressionless face with wasting of temporalis, masseters and sternomastoids, diabetes mellitus, dysphagia due to oesophageal involvement, low IQ, gynaecomastia, testicular atrophy, cardiomyopathy, respiratory infection and somnolence. Myotonia is the continued contraction of the muscle after voluntary contraction ceases, followed by impaired relaxation (often noticed when shaking hands with the patient).

278. A. T   B. F   C. F   D. T   E. T

In myasthenia gravis, edrophonium often produces temporary improvement of muscle strength and is used to confirm the diagnosis. The electromyogram shows that the muscle action potential produces a decremental response to repetitive nerve stimulation, unlike Eaton–Lambert syndrome and botulism where the response is incremental. Virtually all patient have antibodies against the acetylcholine receptor. Anticholinesterase drugs improve symptoms in these patients. Thymectomy is effective treatment for generalised or disabling ocular myasthenia gravis. Plasmapheresis is used in the treatment of acute exacerbations, although benefits are temporary.

279. A. T   B. T   C. T   D. T   E. F

In Guillain–Barré syndrome the typical presentation is rapidly progressive ascending paralysis and the CSF protein is elevated without increase in cell number. Rapidly progressive muscle weakness may be a presenting feature of polymyositis. Botulism is due to the ingestion of an exotoxin produced by *Clostridium botulinum* that interferes with release of acetylcholine from the presynaptic nerve terminals at the neuromuscular junction. It is characterised by autonomic dysfunction, cranial nerve palsies and weakness. Tetanus is caused by an exotoxin formed by *Clostridium tetani* and causes generalised or localised muscle spasm.

280. *The following statements about Parkinson's disease are correct.*

   A. When tremor is the main problem, anticholinergic drugs should be avoided.
   B. When bradykinesia is the main problem, L-dopa should be avoided.
   C. Drug holidays enhance the efficacy of treatment.
   D. High-protein diets should be avoided in those who have episodes of sudden and substantial loss of mobility.
   E. Tocopherol retards progression of early disease.

   A.......... B.......... C.......... D.......... E..........

281. *The following associations are correct.*

   A. Chorea is associated with degeneration of the caudate nuclei.
   B. Athetosis is associated with lesions in the lenticular nucleus.
   C. Hemiballism is associated with lesions of the subthalamic nuclei.
   D. Huntington's disease is associated with loss of cholinergic and γ-aminobutyric acid (GABA) secreting neurones in the striatum.
   E. Parkinson's disease is associated with degeneration of the dopaminergic neurones in the nigrostriatal system.

   A.......... B.......... C.......... D.......... E..........

282. *The following statements about chronic pain are correct.*

   A. It is the persistence of pain for 3 months or longer.
   B. Hyperactivity of the autonomic nervous system increases in chronic pain.
   C. It leads to significant changes in personality.
   D. Baseline pain refers to the average pain intensity expressed for 12 or more hours in a 24-h period.
   E. Breakthrough pain is transient increase in pain.

   A.......... B.......... C.......... D.......... E..........

283. *The following statements about the management of pain are correct.*

   A. Do not believe the patient's complaint of pain if he or she has multiple pain complaints.
   B. Non-opioid analgesics have a ceiling effect.
   C. Combining opioids with an amphetamine is not desirable.
   D. Tolerance to the respiratory depressive effects of opioids develops rapidly.
   E. Opioids have anti-emetic properties.

   A.......... B.......... C.......... D.......... E..........

280.   A. F   B. F   C. F   D. T   E. F

When tremor is the main problem, anticholinergic drugs such as trihexphenidyl and benztropine are therapy of first choice if no contraindications are present. When bradykinesia is the main problem, L-dopa along with carbidopa is the preferred therapy. Drug holidays were said to enhance efficacy of treatment but recently have shown to be associated with increased mortality. High-protein diets should be avoided because a large influx of dietary amino acids can interfere with the transport of L-dopa into the brain. Tocopherol is of no benefit in Parkinson's disease.

281.   A. T   B. T   C. T   D. T   E. T

Chorea is associated with degeneration of the caudate nuclei, whereas athetosis is due to lesions in the lenticular nuclei. Hemiballism is due to damage of the subthalamic nuclei, whereas Huntington's disease is associated with loss of cholinergic and GABA-secreting neurones in the striatum. Parkinson's disease is associated with degeneration of the dopaminergic neurones of the nigrostriatal system. The term 'basal ganglia' is generally applied to the caudate nucleus, putamen and globus pallidus, three nuclear masses underlying the cortical mantle. The caudate nucleus and putamen are sometimes called the striatum, whereas the putamen and globus pallidus are sometimes called the lenticular nucleus. Functionally these are related to the subthalamic nucleus of Luys and substantia nigra on each side.

282.   A. T   B. F   C. T   D. T   E. T

Chronic pain is the persistence of pain for 3 months or longer. The hyperactivity of the autonomic nervous system of acute pain disappears with adaptation. Chronic pain leads to significant changes in the patient's lifestyle, personality and ability, resulting in an alteration of the patient's quality of life. Baseline pain refers to the average pain intensity expressed for 12 or more hours in a 24-h period. Breakthrough pain is transient increase in pain resulting from voluntary (such as incident pain on movement) and involuntary factors (such as flatulence).

283.   A. F   B. T   C. F   D. T   E. F

Always believe the patient's complaint of pain. Multiple pains are common in patients with advanced disease and need to be prioritised and classified. Non-opioid analgesics have a ceiling effect. Long-term therapy with NSAIDs results in gastrointestinal, renal and haematological side-effects. Without increasing the opioid dose, pain relief can be improved by combining with other drugs including dextroamphetamine, antihistamine (hydroxyzine) or non-opioid analgesics (such as aspirin, paracetamol or ibuprofen). Diazepam and chlorpromazine do not provide additive analgesic effect, but instead may increase sedation. Tolerance to the respiratory depressive effects of opioids develops rapidly, allowing escalation of dose and prolonged therapy. Opioids have emetic properties and may have to be combined with anti-emetics to prevent this side-effect. Tolerance also rapidly develops to the emetic effect of opioids, allowing discontinuation of anti-emetics.

284. *The following statements about opioid tolerance are correct.*

A. Increased opioid requirements are more commonly associated with tolerance rather than disease progression.
B. Because the analgesic effect is a logarithmic function of the dose of the opioid, doubling the dose may be needed to restore the analgesic effect.
C. Cross-tolerance among opioid analgesics is complete, therefore disallowing a change to an alternative opioid.
D. Tolerance is characterised by the appearance of withdrawal signs similar to those which appear on abrupt withdrawal of the drug.
E. Tolerance is common in patients receiving opioid analgesics chronically for pain.

A.......... B.......... C.......... D.......... E..........

285. *The following statements about adjuvant analgesics are correct.*

A. Caffeine improves the analgesic effects of opioids.
B. Carbamazepine is useful in lancinating pains.
C. Methotrimeprazine, a phenothiazine, has an analgesic potential close to morphine.
D. Corticosteroids ameliorate pain in patients with bone metastases.
E. Tricyclic antidepressants are useful in neuropathic pain.

A.......... B.......... C.......... D.......... E..........

286. *The following statements about neurosurgical approaches to improve pain are correct.*

A. Cordotomy for unilateral pain below the waist is contraindicated in cancer patients with a relatively short life expectancy.
B. Dorsal rhizotomy is the procedure commonly used in patients with chest wall pain from tumour invasion.
C. Transcutaneous electrical nerve stimulation is used in intractable deafferentation pain.
D. Cordotomy involves interrupting ascending spinothalamic tracts.
E. Cordotomy is particularly useful in patients with chest wall or upper extremity involvement.

A.......... B.......... C.......... D.......... E..........

287. *Recognised causes of predominantly motor neuropathy include*

A. lead toxicity.
B. peroneal muscular atrophy.
C. porphyria.
D. organophosphorous poisoning.
E. dapsone toxicity.

A.......... B.......... C.......... D.......... E..........

284. A. F   B. T   C. F   D. F   E. T

Tolerance is common in patients receiving opioid analgesics chronically for pain. Increased opioid requirements are more commonly associated with disease progression rather than drug tolerance. Because the analgesic effect is a logarithmic function of the dose of the opioid, doubling the dose may be needed to restore the analgesic effect. Cross-tolerance among opioid analgesics is incomplete, therefore allowing a change to an alternative opioid at a starting dose of one-quarter to one-half of the predicted equianalgesic dose. Physical and psychological dependence are distinct from tolerance. Physical dependence is characterised by the appearance of withdrawal signs on abruptly withdrawing the opioid.

285. A. T   B. T   C. T   D. T   E. T

Psychostimulants such as caffeine and dextroamphetamine are effective in improving opioid-induced analgesia and the latter also counteracts opioid-induced sedation. Carbamazepine, baclofen and pimozide are useful in lancinating pains. Methotrimeprazine, a phenothiazine, has an analgesic potential close to morphine. Corticosteroids ameliorate pain, improve appetite and reduce nausea in patients with bone metastases from breast or prostate cancer. Tricyclic antidepressants are useful in neuropathic pain.

286. A. F   B. T   C. T   D. T   E. F

Cordotomy involves interrupting ascending spinothalamic tracts. Cordotomy is the procedure of choice for unilateral pain below the waist in cancer patients with a relatively short life expectancy. Although cordotomy is initially useful in chest wall or upper extremity pain, the level of analgesia falls with time, limiting the usefulness of this approach. Dorsal rhizotomy is the procedure commonly used in patients with chest wall pain from tumour invasion and ameliorates pain in 80% of patients treated. Transcutaneous electrical nerve stimulation is used in intractable deafferentation and dysaesthetic pain.

287. A. T   B. T   C. T   D. T   E. T

Causes of predominantly motor neuropathy include Guillain–Barré syndrome, peroneal muscular atrophy, lead toxicity, porphyria, dapsone toxicity and organophosphorous poisoning.

288. *Causes of predominantly sensory neuropathy include*

    A. diabetes mellitus.
    B. alcoholism.
    C. chronic renal failure.
    D. Guillain–Barré syndrome.
    E. leprosy.

    A.......... B.......... C.......... D.......... E..........

289. *Causes of mononeuritis multiplex include*

    A. diabetes mellitus.
    B. systemic lupus erythematosus.
    C. polyarteritis nodosa.
    D. leprosy.
    E. rheumatoid arthritis.

    A.......... B.......... C.......... D.......... E..........

290. *Causes of thickened nerves include*

    A. amyloidosis.
    B. Charcot–Marie–Tooth disease.
    C. autonomic neuropathy.
    D. Refsum's disease.
    E. Déjérine–Sottas disease.

    A.......... B.......... C.......... D.......... E..........

291. *Recognised features of Charcot–Marie–Tooth disease include*

    A. pes cavus.
    B. inverted champagne bottle legs.
    C. foot-drop.
    D. retinitis pigmentosa.
    E. wasting of the small muscles of the hand.

    A.......... B.......... C.......... D.......... E..........

292. *Recognised causes of bilateral wasted hands include*

    A. rheumatoid arthritis.
    B. motor neurone disease.
    C. cervical spondylosis.
    D. Pancoast's tumour.
    E. old age.

    A.......... B.......... C.......... D.......... E..........

288. A. T   B. T   C. T   D. F   E. T

Causes of predominantly sensory neuropathy include diabetes mellitus, alcoholism, chronic renal failure and deficiencies of vitamin B_{12} and B_1.

289. A. T   B. T   C. T   D. T   E. T

Causes of mononeuritis multiplex include Wegener's granulomatosis, amyloidosis, rheumatoid arthritis, diabetes mellitus, systemic lupus erythematosus, polyarteritis nodosa, leprosy, carcinomatosis, Churg–Strauss syndrome (mnemonic: WARDS, PLC).

290. A. T   B. T   C. T   D. T   E. T

Causes of thickened nerves include amyloidosis, Charcot–Marie–Tooth disease, leprosy, Refsum's disease and Déjérine–Sottas disease.

291. A. T   B. T   C. T   D. T   E. T

Charcot–Marie–Tooth disease has three recognised forms: (1) hereditary motor sensory neuropathy (HMSN) type I with dominant inheritance, which is a demyelinating neuropathy; (2) HMSN type II, an axonal neuropathy; and (3) distal spinal muscular atrophy. Recognised clinical features include wasting of the small muscles of the hands, pes cavus, high-stepping gait of foot-drop, thickened greater auricular nerves and lateral popliteal nerves, scoliosis of the spine, optic atrophy, retinitis pigmentosa and spastic paraparesis.

292. A. T   B. T   C. T   D. F   E. T

Causes of bilateral wasted hands include rheumatoid arthritis, old age, cervical spondylosis, bilateral cervical ribs, bilateral median and ulnar nerve lesions, motor neurone disease, syringomyelia, Charcot–Marie–Tooth disease and Guillain–Barré syndrome. Unilateral wasting of the hand is seen in Pancoast's tumour and brachial plexus trauma.

293. *Causes of proximal muscle weakness with normal serum CK levels include*

A. steroids
B. polymyositis.
C. lovastatin.
D. chloroquine.
E. colchicine.

A........... B.......... C.......... D.......... E..........

294. *Recognised manifestations of Landouzy–Déjérine syndrome include*

A. markedly reduced lifespan.
B. elevated serum CK levels.
C. winging of the scapula.
D. low IQ.
E. autosomal recessive inheritance.

A........... B.......... C.......... D.......... E..........

295. *Recognised clinical features of Friedreich's ataxia include*

A. pes cavus.
B. pyramidal weakness in the legs.
C. cerebellar signs.
D. impaired vibration and joint sense.
E. distal muscle wasting.

A........... B.......... C.......... D.......... E..........

296. *Conditions in which there is absent knee jerk with upgoing plantar (Babinski) response include*

A. the absence of peripheral neuropathy in a stroke patient.
B. motor neurone disease.
C. tabes dorsalis.
D. subacute combined degeneration of the spinal cord.
E. Friedreich's ataxia.

A........... B.......... C.......... D.......... E..........

297. *Recognised features of motor neurone disease include the following:*

A. it usually begins before the second decade.
B. sensory symptoms are prominent.
C. ocular movements are severely affected.
D. cerebellar signs are prominent.
E. sphincters are involved early in the course of the disease in most patients.

A........... B.......... C.......... D.......... E..........

293. A. T   B. F   C. F   D. F   E. F

Proximal muscle weakness with high serum CK levels is seen in polymyositis, lovastatin, chloroquine and colchicine therapy and in patients on chronic haemodialysis. Steroids cause proximal muscle weakness with normal serum CK levels.

294. A. F   B. F   C. T   D. F   E. F

Landouzy–Déjérine syndrome (facioscapulohumeral dystrophy) is an autosomal dominant disorder that affects both sexes between the age of 10 and 40 years. Patients have a normal IQ, normal lifespan and normal muscle enzymes. Other features include ptosis, marked facial weakness, impaired speech, wasting of the sternomastoids and marked weakness of neck muscles, winging of scapula, weakness of lower pectorals and lower trapezii, weakness of triceps and biceps, true hypertrophy of deltoids to compensate for other muscles and absent biceps and triceps jerk.

295. A. T   B. T   C. T   D. T   E. T

Clinical features of Friedreich's ataxia include kyphoscoliosis, pes cavus and a combination of pyramidal, cerebellar and sensory deficits in the lower limbs, hypertrophic cardiomyopathy, optic atrophy (in one-third of cases), diabetes (in 10%) and intellectual deterioration.

296. A. F   B. T   C. T   D. T   E. T

Conditions with absent knee jerk and upgoing plantar response include peripheral neuropathy in a stroke patient, motor neurone disease, conus medullaris–cauda equina lesion, tabes dorsalis and subacute combined degeneration of the spinal cord.

297. A. F   B. F   C. F   D. F   E. F

Characteristic features of motor neurone disease include the following: it rarely begins before the age of 40 years, there is upper and lower motor neurone involvement of a single spinal segment and motor dysfunction involving at least two limbs or one limb and bulbar muscles, sensory symptoms or signs are not seen, ocular movements are not affected, there are never cerebellar or extrapyramidal signs, sphincters are involved late if at all, and remission is unknown and the disease is usually fatal within 5 years (due to bronchopneumonia).

298. *Abnormalities associated with neurofibroma include*

A. lung cysts.
B. pseudoarthrosis of the tibia.
C. aqueductal stenosis.
D. epilepsy.
E. rib notching.

A........... B.......... C.......... D.......... E..........

299. *Recognised causes of dissociated sensory loss include*

A. anterior spinal artery occlusion.
B. diabetic small-fibre polyneuropathy.
C. leprosy.
D. syringomyelia.
E. hereditary amyloidotic polyneuropathy.

A........... B.......... C.......... D.......... E..........

300. *The Wasserman reaction for syphilis is positive in*

A. rheumatoid arthritis.
B. systemic lupus erythematosus.
C. chronic active hepatitis.
D. infectious mononucleosis.
E. general paralysis of the insane.

A........... B.......... C.......... D.......... E..........

301. *Recognised features of ulnar nerve palsy include*

A. wasting of the muscles of the upper arm above the elbow.
B. wasting of small muscles of the hand.
C. sensory loss over the lateral one and a half fingers.
D. weakness of the muscles of the thenar eminence.
E. claw hand.

A........... B.......... C.......... D.......... E..........

302. *Causes of claw hand include*

A. leprosy.
B. advanced rheumatoid arthritis.
C. syringomyelia.
D. Klumpke's paralysis.
E. lesions of the medial cord of the brachial plexus.

A........... B.......... C.......... D.......... E..........

298. A. T   B. T   C. T   D. T   E. T

Abnormalities associated with neurofibroma include lung cysts, retinal hamartomas, skeletal lesions including rib notching, intraosseous cystic lesions, subperiosteal bone cysts, dysplasia of the skull, bowed legs and pseudoarthrosis of the tibia, intellectual disability, epilepsy and sarcomatous change.

299. A. T   B. T   C. T   D. T   E. T

Dissociated sensory loss is the loss of pain and temperature sensation with intact vibration, light touch and joint position sense. It is seen in syringomyelia, anterior spinal artery occlusion (affecting the dorsal horn and lateral spinothalamic tract) and conditions that affect small peripheral nerve axons (including diabetic small-fibre polyneuropathy, hereditary amyloidotic polyneuropathy and leprosy).

300. A. T   B. T   C. T   D. T   E. T

The Wasserman reaction for syphilis is falsely positive in rheumatoid arthritis, systemic lupus erythematosus, chronic active hepatitis and infectious mononucleosis. It is positive in 100% of patients with general paralysis of the insane, in 75% of patients with tabes dorsalis and 70% of patients with meningovascular syphilis.

301. A. F   B. T   C. F   D. F   E. T

The ulnar nerve is derived from the eighth cervical and first thoracic spinal nerves. It has no branches above the elbow and supplies the flexor carpi ulnaris and medial half of the flexor digitorum profundus in the forearm, in the hand it supplies muscles of the little finger, adductor pollicis, interossei, third and fourth lumbricals, palmaris brevis and inner head of the flexor pollicis brevis. Ulnar nerve palsy causes generalised wasting of the small muscles of the hand, weakness of movement of the fingers except that of the thenar eminence, and sensory loss over the medial one and a half fingers. It causes the ulnar claw hand, i.e. hyperextension at the metacarpophalangeal joints and flexion at the interphalangeal joints of the fourth and fifth fingers. The index and middle fingers are less affected as the first and second lumbricals are supplied by the median nerve.

302. A. T   B. T   C. T   D. T   E. T

True claw hand is seen in the following conditions: advanced rheumatoid arthritis, lesions of both the median and ulnar nerves as in leprosy, lesions of the medial cord of the brachial plexus, anterior poliomyelitis, syringomyelia, polyneuritis, amyotrophic lateral sclerosis, Klumpke's paralysis (lower brachial plexus, C7–C8 involvement) and severe Volkmann's ischaemic contracture.

303. *The following statements about nerve injury are correct.*

A. In neuropraxia, recovery does not occur.
B. Axonotmesis is when the nerve is completely severed.
C. Neurotmesis is a concussion of the nerve.
D. In neurotmesis, the prognosis for complete recovery is excellent.
E. In axonotmesis recovery may occur.

A............   B...........   C...........   D...........   E...........

304. *Causes of foot-drop include*

A. common peroneal nerve palsy.
B. root lesions of the first and second lumbar segments.
C. motor neurone disease.
D. lumbosacral plexus lesion.
E. sciatic nerve palsy.

A............   B...........   C...........   D...........   E...........

305. *Recognised causes of carpal tunnel syndrome include*

A. thyrotoxicosis.
B. pregnancy.
C. acromegaly.
D. rheumatoid arthritis.
E. patients on long-term haemodialysis.

A............   B...........   C...........   D...........   E...........

306. *Causes of internuclear ophthalmoplegia include*

A. damage to the second cranial nerve.
B. multiple sclerosis.
C. pontine glioma.
D. inflammatory lesions of the brainstem.
E. trauma to the cervical spinal cord.

A............   B...........   C...........   D...........   E...........

307. *Causes of cerebellopontine angle lesions include*

A. acoustic neuroma.
B. medulloblastoma of the cerebellum.
C. carcinoma of nasopharynx.
D. aneurysm of the basilar artery.
E. local meningeal involvement by tuberculosis.

A............   B...........   C...........   D...........   E...........

303. A. F   B. F   C. F   D. F   E. T

Neuropraxia is concussion of the nerve, after which complete recovery occurs. In axonotmesis, in which the axon is severed but the myelin sheath is intact, recovery may occur. In neurotmesis, the nerve is completely severed and the prognosis for recovery is poor.

304. A. T   B. F   C. T   D. T   E. T

Causes of foot-drop include peripheral neuropathy, L4–L5 root lesion, motor neurone disease, sciatic nerve palsy and lumbosacral plexus lesion.

305. A. F   B. T   C. T   D. T   E. T

Carpal tunnel syndrome is due to median nerve involvement in the hand, resulting in wasting of the thenar eminence, weakness of flexion, abduction and opposition of the thumb and diminished sensation over the lateral three and a half fingers. Causes include pregnancy, oral contraceptives, rheumatoid arthritis, myxoedema, acromegaly, chronic renal failure patients on long-term haemodialysis, sarcoidosis and hyperparathyroidism.

306. A. F   B. T   C. T   D. T   E. F

Internuclear ophthalmoplegia is due to a lesion in the medial longitudinal bundle in the brainstem, which connects the sixth cranial nerve nucleus on one side to the third nerve nucleus on the opposite side of the brainstem. The eye will not adduct because the third nerve, and therefore the medial rectus, have been disconnected from the lateral gaze centre and sixth nerve nucleus of the opposite side. Nystagmus is more prominent in the abducting eye and the patient has a divergent squint. Causes include multiple sclerosis, vascular disease, pontine glioma and inflammatory lesions of the brainstem.

307. A. T   B. T   C. T   D. T   E. T

The cerebellopontine angle is a shallow triangular fossa lying between the cerebellum, lateral pons and the inner third of the petrous temporal bone. It extends from the trigeminal nerve (above) to the glossopharyngeal nerve (below). The abducens nerve runs along the medial edge, whereas the facial and auditory cranial nerves traverse the angle to enter the internal auditory meatus. Damage to the seventh and eighth cranial nerves is the hallmark of a lesion in this region. Cerebellar signs and loss of corneal reflex and trigeminal nerve involvement are other features. Causes of cerebellopontine angle lesions include acoustic neuroma, meningioma, cholesteatoma, haemangioblastoma, aneurysm of the basilar artery, pontine glioma, medulloblastoma and astrocytoma of the cerebellum, carcinoma of the nasopharynx and local meningeal involvement by syphilis and tuberculosis.

308. *The following associations are correct.*

    A. Fifth cervical root lesion is associated with sensory deficit of the ring and little fingers.

    B. Seventh cervical root lesion is associated with weakness of the triceps.

    C. Sixth cervical root lesion is associated with diminished biceps jerk.

    D. Eighth cervical root lesion is associated with weakness of the deltoids.

    E. First thoracic root lesion is associated with weakness of the small muscles of the hand.

    A........... B.......... C.......... D.......... E..........

309. *The following statements about dementia are correct.*

    A. Alzheimer's dementia comprises less than 10% of all causes of dementia.

    B. Multi-infarct dementia is reserved for patients with compelling stroke-like clinical and radiographic features.

    C. Alcohol abuse causes dementia in many ways.

    D. Depression causes pseudodementia.

    E. Dementia is often associated with neurodegenerative disorders.

    A........... B.......... C.......... D.......... E..........

310. *Causes of optic atrophy include*

    A. multiple sclerosis.

    B. glaucoma.

    C. Friedreich's ataxia.

    D. Paget's disease.

    E. secondary to retinitis pigmentosa.

    A........... B.......... C.......... D.......... E..........

308.   A. F   B. T   C. T   D. F   E. T

Seventh cervical root lesion causes weakness of the triceps, fifth cervical root lesion results in weakness of the deltoids, sixth cervical root lesion results in diminished biceps jerk, eighth cervical root lesion causes sensory deficit of the ring and little fingers and first thoracic root lesion causes weakness of the small muscles of the hand.

309.   A. F   B. T   C. T   D. T   E. T

Alzheimer's dementia comprises over half of all causes of dementia. Multi-infarct dementia should be reserved for patients with compelling stroke-like clinical and radiographic features. Alcohol abuse causes dementia in many ways, including recurrent head trauma, vitamin deficiencies, direct neurotoxicity and coagulopathies leading to subdural haematomas. Depression causes pseudodementia and often an empirical trial of antidepressant medication may be beneficial. Dementia is often associated with neurodegenerative disorders including Parkinson's disease, progressive supranuclear palsy and Huntington's disease.

310.   A. T   B. T   C. T   D. T   E. T

All are true.

8   NEPHROLOGY

311.   *The following associations about urinary findings are correct.*

   A. Granular casts–ischaemic damage of the tubules.
   B. WBC casts–pyelonephritis.
   C. Red blood cell casts–glomerulonephritis.
   D. Epithelial cells–ischaemic damage of the tubules.
   E. Massive proteinuria–nephrotic syndrome.

   A..........   B..........   C..........   D..........   E..........

312.   *The following statements about urinary tract infections (UTIs) are correct.*

   A. Acute uncomplicated cystitis in women is caused by *E. coli* in less than 10% of cases.
   B. Recurrent cystitis in a young woman is usually due to urological abnormalities.
   C. Acute uncomplicated pyelonephritis in young women is usually due to *E. coli.*
   D. UTIs are common in men younger than 50 years.
   E. Urinary catheter-associated bacteriuria is the most common source of Gram-negative bacteraemia in hospitalised patients.

   A..........   B..........   C..........   D..........   E..........

313.   *The following statements are correct.*

   A. Asymptomatic bacteriuria is defined as two successive cultures with greater than or equal to 10^5 colony-forming units per millilitre.
   B. Acute urethral syndrome is a condition of women who have lower urinary tract symptoms and pyuria with fewer than 10^5 bacteria per millilitre of urine.
   C. Prostatitis is usually caused by Gram-positive cocci.
   D. Epididymitis is usually caused by *N. gonorrhoeae* or *Chl. trachomatis* in sexually active young women.
   E. Epididymitis in older men is usually caused by Gram-positive organisms.

   A..........   B..........   C..........   D..........   E..........

311. A. T   B. T   C. T   D. T   E. T

The presence of epithelial cells and granular casts with a dirty brown sediment indicate ischaemic renal damage. WBC casts are seen in pyelonephritis, whereas red blood cell casts are a feature of glomerulonephritis. Massive proteinuria is the cardinal feature of nephrotic syndrome.

312. A. F   B. F   C. T   D. F   E. T

Acute uncomplicated cystitis in women is caused by *E. coli* in 80% of cases. Recurrent cystitis in a young woman is usually due to reinfection and is rarely a result of abnormalities of the urinary tract. Acute uncomplicated pyelonephritis in young women is usually due to *E. coli*. UTIs are rare in men younger than 50 years, however, it does not necessarily mean urological abnormalities. Urinary catheter-associated bacteriuria is the most common source of Gram-negative bacteraemia in hospitalised patients; therefore, urinary catheters should be used only when absolutely necessary.

313. A. T   B. T   C. F   D. T   E. F

Asymptomatic bacteriuria is defined as two successive cultures with greater than or equal to 10^5 colony-forming units per millilitre. Acute urethral syndrome is a condition of women who have lower urinary tract symptoms and pyuria with fewer than 10^5 bacteria per millilitre of urine. Prostatitis is usually caused by Gram-negative enteric cocci. Epididymitis is usually caused by *N. gonorrhoeae* or *Chl. trachomatis* in sexually active young women. Epididymitis in older men is usually caused by Gram-positive organisms.

314. *The following statements are correct.*

    A. When the glomerular filtration rate is markedly reduced, the measurement of creatine clearance may actually underestimate the true rate.

    B. Small kidneys generally indicate chronic renal disease.

    C. Radionuclide renal scan is useful when there is an anomaly of renal blood flow.

    D. Renal biopsy is contraindicated in systemic lupus erythematosus.

    E. MRI is useful in the evaluation of atherosclerosis of the proximal renal arteries.

    A..........   B..........   C..........   D..........   E..........

315. *The following statements about prerenal azotaemia are correct.*

    A. It is a disorder that results from an increase in effective arterial blood volume.

    B. The fractional excretion of sodium is usually less than 1%.

    C. Fluid challenge is contraindicated in oliguric patients even when they are not volume overloaded

    D. Diuretic treatment may convert oliguric renal failure to non-oliguric renal failure.

    E. Dopamine therapy is contraindicated in these patients.

    A..........   B..........   C..........   D..........   E..........

316. *The following associations are correct.*

    A. Radiocontrast nephropathy–long-standing diabetes mellitus.

    B. Aminoglycoside nephropathy–damage of proximal tubules.

    C. Pigment-induced renal damage–cytotoxic therapy of haematological malignancies.

    D. Acute uric acid nephropathy–rhabdomyolysis.

    E. Allergic interstitial nephritis–eosinophilia.

    A..........   B..........   C..........   D..........   E..........

317. *Management of oliguric acute renal failure includes the following:*

    A. daily protein intake should be increased to $1.5\,g\,kg^{-1}$.

    B. daily potassium intake should be restricted to 40 mEq.

    C. antihypertensive medications that do not decrease renal blood flow are preferred.

    D. mild elevations of serum uric acid do not require treatment.

    E. Anaemia should be treated with erythropoietin.

    A..........   B..........   C..........   D..........   E..........

314. A. F   B. T   C. T   D. F   E. T

When the glomerular filtration rate is markedly reduced, the measurement of creatine clearance may actually overestimate the true rate. Small kidneys indicate chronic renal disease, although the kidneys may be enlarged when the underlying cause is diabetes, amyloidosis or multiple myeloma. Radionuclide renal scan is useful when there is an anomaly of renal blood flow. Renal biopsy is useful in the evaluation of patients with proteinuria, haematuria or casts. It is useful in obtaining prognostic information in the evaluation of systemic lupus erythematosus. MRI scans are useful in the evaluation of atherosclerosis of the proximal renal arteries or renal masses.

315. A. F   B. T   C. F   D. T   E. F

Prerenal azotaemia results from a decrease in effective arterial blood volume. The kidney attempts to reabsorb filtered sodium and the fractional excretion of sodium is usually less than 1%. Patients who are oliguric and not fluid overloaded may benefit from a fluid challenge. The addition of diuretics such as metolazone, frusemide and mannitol may convert oliguric renal failure to non-oliguric renal failure and improve prognosis. Dopamine may be effective at low doses, when it improves renal blood flow and results in diuresis.

316. A. T   B. T   C. F   D. F   E. T

Long-standing diabetes mellitus, heart failure, pre-existing renal insufficiency, age greater than 70 years and multiple myeloma are said to be risk factors for radiocontrast nephropathy. Aminoglycosides cause toxicity of the proximal tubules and often cause non-oliguric renal failure. Rhabdomyolysis and haemolysis cause pigment-induced renal damage. Intratubular precipitation of uric acid and the consequent renal failure occurs as a result of cell lysis due to cytotoxic therapy for haematological malignancies. Allergic interstitial nephritis is associated with penicillins, NSAIDs and sulphonamides and usually resolves with discontinuation of the offending drug. Accompanying features include eosinophilia, elevated serum IgE and eosinophiluria.

317. A. F   B. T   C. T   D. T   E. F

Daily protein and potassium intake should be restricted $0.5\,\mathrm{g\,kg}^{-1}$ and 40 mEq respectively. Treatment of blood pressure is best done with drugs that do not decrease renal blood flow, e.g. calcium channel blockers, prazosin or clonidine. Mild elevations of serum uric acid are frequent in acute renal failure and do not require treatment unless they are markedly elevated, when allopurinol should be added to the drug regimen. Erythropoietin is not effective in the short-term management of anaemia.

318. *Indications for dialysis in acute renal failure include*

A. severe hyperkalaemia.
B. severe acidosis.
C. marked volume overload.
D. uraemic pericarditis.
E. encephalopathy.

A........... B.......... C.......... D.......... E..........

319. *The following statements about minimal change glomerular disease are correct.*

A. It presents with nephrotic syndrome.
B. Failure to respond to steroids may reflect an error in diagnosis.
C. Progression to chronic renal failure is common.
D. It is associated with Hodgkin's disease.
E. Relapses are usually resistant to steroid therapy.

A........... B.......... C.......... D.......... E..........

320. *The following statements about glomerular disease are correct.*

A. Focal segmental glomerular sclerosis rapidly progresses to renal failure.
B. Biopsy in membranous glomerulonephropathy shows thickening of the glomerular capillary wall secondary to subepithelial deposits of IgG and C3.
C. Serum complement levels are low in membranoproliferative glomerulonephropathy.
D. The majority of patients with idiopathic rapidly progressive glomerulonephritis are resistant to glucocorticoid therapy.
E. Plasmapheresis is contraindicated when the kidney is affected in Goodpasture's syndrome.

A........... B.......... C.......... D.......... E..........

321. *Causes of nephrotic syndrome include*

A. coronary artery disease.
B. diabetes mellitus.
C. systemic lupus erythematosus.
D. amyloidosis.
E. multiple myeloma.

A........... B.......... C.......... D.......... E..........

322. *The management of nephrotic syndrome includes*

A. avoidance of diuretics to treat oedema.
B. ACE inhibitors.
C. hepatic HMG-CoA reductase inhibitors.
D. dietary protein restriction in those with renal insufficiency.
E. prophylactic anticoagulants in all patients.

A........... B.......... C.......... D.......... E..........

318.   A. T   B. T   C. T   D. T   E. T

Indications for dialysis in acute renal failure include severe acidosis, hyperkalaemia or marked fluid overload resistant to conventional therapy, uraemic pericarditis and encephalopathy (lethargy, seizures, myoclonus and asterixis).

319.   A. T   B. T   C. F   D. T   E. F

Minimal change glomerular disease is a pathological diagnosis that includes normal light microscopy, negative immunofluorescence and fusion of foot processes on electron microscopy. These patients present with nephrotic syndrome and usually respond to steroid therapy; failure to respond may reflect an error in diagnosis. Relapses often respond to reinstitution of steroid therapy. Both Hodgkin's and non-Hodgkin's lymphomas are associated with this disease.

320.   A. F   B. T   C. T   D. F   E. F

Focal segmental glomerular sclerosis slowly progresses to chronic renal failure about 5–10 years after first diagnosis. Renal biopsy in membranous glomerulonephropathy shows thickening of the glomerular capillary wall secondary to subepithelial deposits of IgG and C3. Serum complement levels are low in membranoproliferative glomerulonephropathy and the diagnosis should be suspected in those with a clinical picture of acute glomerulonephritis or nephrotic syndrome. The majority of patients with idiopathic rapidly progressive glomerulonephritis respond to pulsed high-dose glucocorticoid therapy. Patients with Goodpasture's syndrome require clearance of antibodies to glomerular basement membrane by plasmapheresis, in addition to the suppression of formation of new antibodies using cyclophosphamide and prednisolone.

321.   A. F   B. T   C. T   D. T   E. T

Causes of nephrotic syndrome include primary glomerular disease, diabetes mellitus, systemic lupus erythematosus, amyloidosis and multiple myeloma.

322.   A. F   B. T   C. T   D. T   E. F

Judicious use of diuretics, including frusemide and metolazone, is effective in the resolution of oedema of nephrotic syndrome. ACE inhibitors reduce proteinuria, particularly in diabetic patients, and are said to have long-term benefits. Hepatic HMG-CoA reductase inhibitors and dietary restriction of saturated fats and cholesterol are used to improve the lipoprotein profile in these patients but the long-term benefits are not clear. Dietary protein restriction is appropriate in those with renal insufficiency; the amount of protein equal to the urinary loss should be added to the calculated protein restriction to compute the total daily intake. Renal vein thrombosis and other thromboembolic complications are common in nephrotic syndrome but long-term anticoagulant therapy is initiated only in those with these complications.

323. *In chronic renal failure*

   A. protein restriction will reduce accumulation of nitrogenous waste products.
   B. there is retention of phosphate.
   C. there is excessive renal loss of magnesium.
   D. correction of anaemia with erythropoietin is not required in those on regular long-term dialysis.
   E. elevated aluminium tissue levels can cause osteomalacia.

   A........... B.......... C.......... D.......... E..........

324. *The following statements about haemodialysis are correct.*

   A. It works by diffusion of high-molecular-weight solutes across a semi-permeable membrane.
   B. When haemodialysis is instituted, daily dietary protein should be decreased to $0.5\,g\,kg^{-1}$.
   C. Dialysis disequilibrium is a syndrome that may occur during the first few treatments of profoundly uraemic patients and is attributed to CNS oedema.
   D. Treatment of pericarditis occurring in patients undergoing dialysis involves intensification of dialysis.
   E. Dialysis dementia is due to depletion of CNS aluminium.

   A........... B.......... C.......... D.......... E..........

325. *The following statements are correct.*

   A. Peritoneal dialysis is contraindicated in diabetic patients.
   B. Haemofiltration removes large amounts of metabolic wastes with minimal removal of fluid.
   C. Cyclosporin is contraindicated in cadaver allograft renal transplants.
   D. Anti-T-lymphocyte monoclonal antibody (OKT3) is used in the management of acute renal graft rejection.
   E. One-year graft survival rates for cadaver renal transplants are higher compared with live-related donor transplants.

   A........... B.......... C.......... D.......... E..........

326. *The following statements about kidney stones are correct.*

   A. Hyperparathyroidism resulting in renal stone formation should be treated with parathyroidectomy.
   B. Uric acid stones account for about 75% of all stones.
   C. Struvite stones are associated with infections due to urea-splitting organisms.
   D. Calcium stones are associated with hyperoxaluria.
   E. Cystine stones arise from an inborn error in amino acid transport.

   A........... B.......... C.......... D.......... E..........

323. A. T   B. T   C. F   D. F   E. T

Protein restriction will reduce accumulation of nitrogenous waste products. This results in the retention of phosphate, resulting in increased serum phosphate and an accompanying fall in serum calcium. The latter two biochemical anomalies are further exacerbated by resistance to parathyroid hormone action on the bone and decreased production of 1,25-dihydroxyvitamin D_3. These changes result in increased parathyroid hormone (secondary hyperparathyroidism), which contributes to renal osteodystrophy. Osteomalacia and aplastic bone disease also occur, usually due to aluminium retention. Definitive diagnosis of aluminium-related bone disease requires bone biopsy. Magnesium is excreted by the kidney and in chronic renal failure accumulation should be avoided by restricting dietary intake.

324. A. F   B. F   C. T   D. T   E. F

Haemodialysis works by diffusion of low-molecular-weight solutes across a semi-permeable membrane. When haemodialysis is instituted, daily dietary protein should be increased to $1-1.2 \, \text{g} \, \text{kg}^{-1}$. Dialysis disequilibrium is a syndrome that may occur during the first few dialyses of profoundly uraemic patients and is attributed to CNS oedema. Treatment of pericarditis occurring in patients undergoing dialysis involves intensification of dialysis to once every day. Dialysis dementia is due to accumulation of CNS aluminium; chelation therapy with desferrioxamine may improve or stop the progression of dementia in some patients.

325. A. F   B. F   C. F   D. T   E. F

Although peritoneal dialysis increases blood sugar levels, appropriate administration of insulin allows this procedure to be carried out in diabetic patients. Haemofiltration and ultrafiltration remove large volumes of fluid with very minimal removal of metabolic wastes and are used to reduce volume and fluid overload. The 1-year graft survival rate for cadaver renal transplant is 80% compared with 90% for live-related donor transplant. The use of cyclosporin has improved survival rates in cadaver transplants. High-dose intravenous methylprednisolone, anti-T-lymphocyte monoclonal antibody (OKT3) and antilymphocyte globulin are used in the management of acute renal graft rejection. There is no specific treatment for chronic rejection.

326. A. T   B. F   C. T   D. T   E. T

Calcium stones form about 80% of all stones. They are composed of calcium oxalate and phosphate and are associated with hypercalciuria, hyperoxaluria, distal renal tubular acidosis, sarcoidosis and medullary sponge kidney. Hyperparathyroidism resulting in renal stone formation should be treated with parathyroidectomy. Struvite stones cause staghorn calculi and are associated with infections due to urea-splitting organisms, particularly *Proteus mirabilis* (which is common when the urinary pH is high). Cystine stones arise from an inborn error in amino acid transport resulting in cystinuria.

327. *The following statements about pregnancy and renal disease are correct.*

    A. An increase in proteinuria with no clinical evidence of toxaemia usually reflects elevated glomerular pressure.
    B. Pregnancy is contraindicated after renal transplantation.
    C. In pregnant women, flare-ups of lupus nephropathy is usually associated with extrarenal manifestations.
    D. Exacerbations of systemic lupus erythematosus during pregnancy may be treated with high dose of steroids, instead of antihypertensives.
    E. ACE inhibitors are the drugs of choice to control hypertensive nephropathy.

    A.......... B.......... C.......... D.......... E..........

328. *Recognised manifestations of polycystic kidney disease include*

    A. autosomal recessive inheritance.
    B. berry aneurysms.
    C. cysts in the liver.
    D. hypertension.
    E. haematuria.

    A.......... B.......... C.......... D.......... E..........

329. *The following statements about renal transplantation are correct.*

    A. Referral for renal transplantation need not be delayed until the patient has begun dialysis.
    B. Human leucocyte antigen (HLA) mismatching has a greater effect on live-related donor transplantation compared with cadaveric kidney transplantation.
    C. Pretreatment of recipients with multiple blood transfusions from the donor tends to increase graft survival.
    D. A positive cross-match by cytotoxicity testing between recipient serum and donor cells is considered to be a contraindication for transplantation.
    E. The 2-year kidney graft survival rate with cadaveric donor transplantation is greater than the survival rate for live related donor transplantation.

    A.......... B.......... C.......... D.......... E..........

330. *Renal cell carcinoma may present as*

    A. fever of unknown origin.
    B. hypercalcaemia.
    C. myopathy
    D. polycythaemia.
    E. Cushing's syndrome.

    A.......... B.......... C.......... D.......... E..........

327. A. T   B. F   C. F   D. T   E. F

An increase in proteinuria with no clinical evidence of toxaemia usually reflects elevated glomerular pressure. Pregnancy is not contra-indicated after renal transplantation. In pregnant women, flare-ups of lupus nephropathy are not associated with extrarenal manifestations. Exacerbations of systemic lupus erythematosus during pregnancy may be treated with high dose of steroids, instead of antihypertensives. ACE inhibitors should be avoided in hypertensive nephropathy.

328. A. F   B. T   C. T   D. T   E. T

Polycystic kidney disease is an autosomal dominant disorder that presents with haematuria, hypertension, urinary tract infection, pain in the lumbar region and uraemic symptoms. Hypertension develops in 75% of cases. Cysts are present in other organs, including the liver (in 30% of cases), spleen, pancreas, lung, ovaries, testes, epididymis, thyroid, uterus, broad ligament and bladder. Subarachnoid haemorrhage from an intracranial berry aneurysm, causing death or neurological lesions, occurs in about 10% of cases.

329. A. T   B. T   C. T   D. T   E. F

Referral for renal transplantation need not be delayed until the patient has begun dialysis. There is some evidence to show that HLA mismatching has a greater effect on live-related donor transplantation compared with cadaveric kidney transplantation. Pretreatment of recipients with multiple blood transfusions from the donor tends to increase graft survival. A positive cross-match by cytotoxicity testing between recipient serum and donor cells is considered to be a contraindication for transplantation. The 2-year kidney graft survival rate with cadaveric donor transplantation is 70%, whereas the survival rate for live related donor transplantation is 85%.

330. A. T   B. T   C. T   D. T   E. T

Renal cell carcinoma has protean manifestations and the classic triad of gross haematuria, flank pain and palpable mass is not common. Most often the tumour presents with systemic symptoms or as an endocrine syndrome. It may present as fever of unknown origin, myopathy, peripheral neuropathy, hypercalcaemia, secondary amyloidosis, congestive heart failure, Cushing's syndrome due to ACTH production, polycythaemia due to increased production of erythropoietin, refractory anaemia, abnormal liver function test, thrombophlebitis, or metastatic lesions in the liver, lung or brain.

331. *Recognised manifestations of Alport's syndrome include*

    A. middle-ear deafness.
    B. more common in females.
    C. posterior cataracts.
    D. defective glomerular basement membrane synthesis.
    E. corneal dystrophy.

    A...........   B..........   C..........   D..........   E..........

331.   A. F   B. F   C. T   D. T   E. T

Alport's syndrome is the name given to the disease in which nephritis is accompanied by nerve deafness and various eye disorders, including lens dislocation, corneal dystrophy and posterior cataracts. Males tend to be affected more frequently and more severely than females and are more likely to progress to renal failure. Defective glomerular basement membrane synthesis underlies the renal lesions.

9 ACID–BASE DISTURBANCES

332. *Recognised features of metabolic alkalosis includes*

   A. a decrease in plasma carbon dioxide.
   B. a reduction in plasma bicarbonate levels.
   C. hypoalbuminaemia.
   D. hyperglycaemia.
   E. hyponatraemia.

   A.......... B.......... C.......... D.......... E..........

333. *The anion gap*

   A. is an indirect measurement of plasma ions not measured by the laboratory.
   B. is defined as the difference between plasma sodium concentration and the sum of the plasma chloride and bicarbonate concentrations.
   C. normally is mostly due to negatively charged plasma proteins.
   D. can decrease in hypoalbuminaemic patients, even in the setting of non-hyperchloraemic metabolic acidosis.
   E. is useful in the diagnosis of respiratory alkalosis.

   A.......... B.......... C.......... D.......... E..........

334. *Recognised features of acute metabolic acidosis include*

   A. increase in respiratory rate.
   B. shallow respiration.
   C. increased susceptibility to cardiac arrhythmias.
   D. increased response to inotropic agents.
   E. loss of calcium from the bone.

   A.......... B.......... C.......... D.......... E..........

335. *Causes of metabolic acidosis include*

   A. Liddle's syndrome.
   B. Bartter's syndrome.
   C. toxic ingestion of methanol.
   D. salicylate overdose.
   E. fistula of the small bowel.

   A.......... B.......... C.......... D.......... E..........

332.   A. F   B. F   C. F   D. F   E. F

Metabolic alkalosis is characterised by an increase in plasma bicarbonate levels. A decrease in plasma carbon dioxide is characteristic of respiratory alkalosis. Hypoalbuminaemia, hyperglycaemia and hyponatraemia may be associated with metabolic alkalosis but are not characteristic features of metabolic alkalosis.

333.   A. T   B. T   C. T   D. T   E. F

The anion gap is an indirect measurement of plasma ions not measured by the laboratory and is useful in the diagnosis of metabolic acidosis. It is defined as the difference between plasma sodium concentration and the sum of the plasma chloride and bicarbonate concentrations. Normally, anion gap is $12 \pm 4\,mEq\,l^{-1}$ and is mostly due to negatively charged plasma proteins. It is elevated in non-hyperchloraemic acidoses, except in the setting of hypoalbuminaemia. Hypoalbuminaemia may decrease anion gap and mask non-hyperchloraemic metabolic acidosis.

334.   A. T   B. F   C. T   D. F   E. F

Acute metabolic acidosis causes deep respiration called Kussmaul breathing. It often increases respiratory rate and metabolic acidosis should be suspected when there is no obvious lung pathology. Patients with metabolic acidosis have an increased susceptibility to cardiac arrhythmias. Cardiac contractility is impaired in these patients and they have a decreased response to inotropes. Loss of calcium from bone occurs in chronic metabolic acidosis.

335.   A. F   B. F   C. T   D. T   E. T

Examples of increased anion-gap acidosis include diabetic ketoacidosis, lactic acidosis, chronic renal failure, alcoholic ketoacidosis, ingestion of methanol or ethylene glycol, alcoholic ketosis, salicylate overdose and starvation. Examples of normal anion-gap acidosis with hyperchloraemia include renal tubular acidosis, gastrointestinal loss of bicarbonate due to fistulas of the small bowel, pancreas or biliary tract, diarrhoea and ureteral diversions. Examples of chloride-responsive alkalosis include loss of gastric acid or diuretic therapy. Chloride-resistant causes of alkalosis include Liddle's syndrome, Bartter's syndrome, Cushing's syndrome and Conn's syndrome.

336.   *The following statements about the management of metabolic acidosis are correct.*

A. Bicarbonate therapy should be withdrawn when the pH reaches 7.2.
B. Shohl's solution is used in those with underlying renal failure.
C. In alcoholic ketoacidosis, both the anion gap and osmolal gap are increased.
D. Treatment of alcoholic ketoacidosis includes replacement of intravenous fluids and glucose.
E. When the pH reaches 7.2, intravenous hydrogen ions should be administered to prevent paradoxical CSF alkalosis.

A............   B..........   C..........   D..........   E..........

337.   *The following statements are correct.*

A. Normally the kidneys compensate for wide variations in sodium intake.
B. The dextrose in intravenous fluids increases the osmolality of the fluid.
C. Lactated Ringer's solution has a composition similar to extracellular fluid.
D. Urinary losses of potassium may occur in the recovery phase of acute tubular necrosis.
E. Rapid internal fluid shifts may occur in peritonitis.

A............   B..........   C..........   D..........   E..........

338.   *Osmolal gap is increased when there is*

A. hypernatraemia.
B. hyperglycaemia.
C. hyperlipidaemia.
D. hyperproteinaemia.
E. increased ethanol ingestion.

A............   B..........   C..........   D..........   E..........

339.   *Hyponatraemia with*

A. an increase in plasma osmolality occurs in hyperglycaemia.
B. a normal plasma osmolality occurs in severe hyperlipidaemia.
C. a decrease in plasma osmolality and in extracellular volume occurs with diuretic therapy.
D. a decrease in plasma osmolality and clinically normal extracellular volume occurs in hysterical polydipsia.
E. an increase in plasma osmolality occurs in hyperproteinaemia.

A............   B..........   C..........   D..........   E..........

336. A. T   B. F   C. T   D. T   E. F

Bicarbonate therapy should be withdrawn when the pH reaches 7.2. Shohl's solution should not be used in those with underlying renal failure. In alcoholic ketoacidosis, both the anion gap and osmolal gap are increased. Treatment of alcoholic ketoacidosis includes replacement of intravenous fluids and glucose. Intravenous hydrogen ions are never used in the management of patients.

337. A. T   B. F   C. T   D. T   E. T

Normal kidneys are capable of compensating for wide variations in sodium intake. The dextrose in intravenous fluid is quickly metabolised into carbon dioxide and water and thus does not affect the osmolality of intravenous fluids. Lactated Ringer's solution is manufactured to simulate extracellular fluid. Urinary losses of potassium may occur in the recovery phase of acute tubular necrosis when there is massive diuresis, with use of diuretics and when there is an excess of mineralocorticoids. Rapid shifts in internal fluid may occur with peritonitis, intestinal obstruction, paralytic ileus, pancreatitis, bacterial enteritis, severe burns and traumatic crush injuries.

338. A. F   B. F   C. T   D. T   E. T

Osmolal gap is increased when there is an excess of unmeasured solutes and occurs when the plasma osmolality exceeds calculated osmolality by more than $10\,\text{mosmol}\,\text{kg}^{-1}$. Calculated osmolality is determined from the most abundant solutes usually present, including sodium, glucose and blood urea nitrogen. Osmolal gap is increased when there is excess of serum lipids, proteins, ethylene glycol, mannitol, ethyl alcohol and other alcohols.

339. A. T   B. T   C. T   D. T   E. F

Hyponatraemia with an increase in plasma osmolality occurs when there is an excess of solutes restricted to the extracellular fluid compartment, as in hyperglycaemia or the use of mannitol in the presence of renal impairment. Treatment is directed toward the correction of hyperglycaemia. Pseudo-hyponatraemia is the presence of hyponatraemia with normal osmolality and is the result of markedly elevated serum lipid levels, as in poorly controlled diabetes mellitus, or hyperproteinaemia as in multiple myeloma. Hyponatraemia with decreased plasma osmolality in the setting of decreased extracellular volume occurs when there is either renal loss (diuretic therapy, polycystic kidney disease, tubulointerstitial diseases) or extrarenal loss (diarrhoea, vomiting, cutaneous loss). Hyponatraemia with decreased plasma osmolality in the setting of normal extracellular volume is seen in hysterical polydipsia (where the urinary osmolality and urinary sodium are low) and in syndrome of inappropriate antidiuretic hormone (SIADH), hypothyroidism, adrenal insufficiency and thiazide diuretic therapy (where the urinary osmolality and urinary sodium are inappropriately excessively high).

340. *Recognised causes of SIADH include*

A. adrenal insufficiency.
B. hypothyroidism.
C. tuberculosis.
D. meningitis.
E. oat cell carcinoma of the lung.

A............   B...........   C...........   D...........   E...........

341. *The following statements about the management of SIADH are correct.*

A. Acute treatment is necessary in patients who are symptomatic or in whom hyponatraemia is severe.
B. Rapid normalisation of sodium levels in chronic SIADH may result in neurological dysfunction.
C. Water restriction should be avoided in the management of chronic SIADH.
D. A loop diuretic is used to lower urine osmolality.
E. The antibiotic demeclocycline is used in the management of chronic SIADH.

A............   B...........   C...........   D...........   E...........

342. *A 60-year-old man has a serum potassium level of $7\,mEq\,l^{-1}$. His ECG may show*

A. peaked T waves.
B. prominent U waves.
C. narrowing of the QRS complex.
D. lengthening of the PR interval.
E. shortened QT interval.

A............   B...........   C...........   D...........   E...........

343. *Recognised causes of hyperkalaemia include*

A. rhabdomyolysis.
B. ACE inhibitors.
C. increased aldosterone production.
D. use of trimethoprim in the treatment of *Pneumocystis carinii* infection in AIDS patients.
E. frusemide therapy.

A............   B...........   C...........   D...........   E...........

340. A. F   B. F   C. T   D. T   E. T

SIADH is a state where patients have euvolaemia with an excess of free water. Consequently it is characterised by hyponatraemia with low plasma osmolality, nearly maximally dilute urine, elevated urinary sodium, normal clinical euvolaemia and normal kidney, thyroid and adrenal function. Recognised causes include neurological conditions (including encephalitis, meningitis, psychosis and intracranial neoplasm), pulmonary causes (tuberculosis, pneumonia, acute asthma, oat cell carcinoma of the lung) and drugs (chlorpropamide, vasopressin, intravenous cyclophosphamide).

341. A. T   B. T   C. F   D. T   E. T

Rapid correction of hyponatraemia is reserved for patients who are symptomatic and in whom the onset of SIADH is acute. In chronic SIADH, rapid correction is not necessary and often results in neurological dysfunction; the mainstay of treatment is water restriction. In patients not responding to water restriction, increasing protein and salt intake is often effective and loop diuretics are used to lower urine osmolality. Demeclocycline is used to antagonise the effect of ADH and is used in chronic treatment.

342. A. T   B. F   C. F   D. T   E. F

When serum potassium is between 5.5 and $6\,\mathrm{mEq\,l^{-1}}$ the ECG shows a shortening of the QT interval and peaking of T waves. Widening of the QRS complex and lengthening of the PR interval occurs at a serum potassium of $6.0–7.0\,\mathrm{mEq\,l^{-1}}$. Further widening of the QRS complex and flattening of the P wave occurs when serum potassium is between 7.0 and $7.5\,\mathrm{mEq\,l^{-1}}$. A biphasic sine wave, which is the result of fusion of widened QRS and T waves is seen when the serum potassium exceeds $8.0\,\mathrm{mEq\,l^{-1}}$ and is a sign of impending ventricular standstill. It must be remembered that the relationship between the level of serum potassium and ECG changes varies from individual to individual and that these ECG changes are less likely to develop when the rise in potassium is slow (as in patients with chronic renal failure). Accompanying electrolyte and acid–base disturbances, as in renal failure, may influence the ECG changes. In hypokalaemia there is T-wave flattening, a decrease in the QRS voltage and ST-segment depression.

343. A. T   B. T   C. F   D. T   E. F

Hyperkalaemia can be caused by (1) diminished renal excretion (as in renal failure), ACE inhibitors, cyclosporin, decreased aldosterone production (as in adrenal insufficiency), impaired response to aldosterone (as with spironolactone therapy) or inhibition of tubular secretion of potassium (e.g. use of trimethoprim in the treatment of *P. carinii* infection in AIDS patients); or (2) excessive potassium due to intravenous administration of potassium or the potassium salt of penicillin, blood transfusion or massive tissue destruction (as in massive burns, rhabdomyolysis, tumour lysis or haemolysis).

344. *A 35-year-old man with polycystic disease and chronic renal failure has a sodium level of*
      140 mEq l⁻¹, a potassium level of 7.0 mEq l⁻¹ and a bicarbonate level of 20 mEq l⁻¹.
      Immediate management includes the following:

   A. administration of intravenous potassium to increase intracellular levels.
   B. glucose and insulin infusions.
   C. avoid administration of intravenous calcium gluconate.
   D. avoid administration of sodium bicarbonate as it causes intracellular
      acidosis.
   E. rectal sodium polystyrene sulphonate.

   A...........   B..........   C..........   D..........   E..........

345. *Causes of respiratory alkalosis include*

   A. hypoventilation.
   B. pregnancy.
   C. Gram–negative sepsis.
   D. pulmonary emboli.
   E. myasthenic crisis.

   A...........   B..........   C..........   D..........   E..........

344. A. F   B. T   C. F   D. F   E. T

This patient has hyperkalaemia and acidosis. Management includes treatment of acidosis and hyperkalaemia. Often, correction of the metabolic acidosis with bicarbonate therapy improves hyperkalaemia by shifting potassium from the extracellular compartment to the intracellular compartment. Similarly, glucose and insulin infusions act to shift potassium from the extracellular fluid into the cells. The β-adrenergic drug albuterol in nebulised form is also useful in treating elevated serum potassium levels in haemodialysis patients by shifting potassium into cells. Polystyrene sulphonate is a cation exchange resin that binds potassium in exchange for sodium in the intestinal tract, thereby removing potassium from the body. Haemodialysis is used when other methods are ineffective or contraindicated.

345. A. F   B. T   C. T   D. T   E. F

Respiratory alkalosis is due to excessive pulmonary carbon dioxde excretion secondary to hyperventilation. Causes include pregnancy, hypoxaemia, drugs (catecholamines, theophyllines, salicylates and progesterone), lung disease (pneumonia, pulmonary emboli, pulmonary oedema and interstitial lung disease), Gram-negative sepsis, hepatic disorders, anxiety, brainstem tumours and excessive mechanical ventilation.

10 RESPIRATORY DISEASES

346. *The following statements about the management of pneumonias are correct.*

    A. Empirical therapy for community-acquired pneumonias should cover for *Strep. pneumoniae.*
    B. Erythromycin is used when *Legionella* is suspected.
    C. Erythromycin is used when *M. pneumoniae* is suspected.
    D. Antibiotics against *Staph. aureus* should be considered during epidemics of influenza.
    E. Nosocomial infection due to *Ps. aeruginosa* is treated with an aminoglycoside and ceftazidime.

    A.......... B.......... C.......... D.......... E..........

347. *A 40-year-old patient comes to the emergency room with an acute exacerbation of bronchial asthma. The following statements about the management are correct.*

    A. The intensity of wheezing is a reliable indicator of severity.
    B. Systemic glucocorticoids speed the resolution of severe exacerbations refractory to bronchodilator therapy.
    C. β-blockers continue to be first-line therapy for rapid symptomatic improvement.
    D. The therapeutic effects of theophylline is not due to bronchodilatation.
    E. Ipratropium bromide is useful in the management of asthma.

    A.......... B.......... C.......... D.......... E..........

348. *Drugs that can exacerbate asthma include*

    A. noradrenaline.
    B. atenolol.
    C. aspirin.
    D. captopril.
    E. inhaled pentamidine.

    A.......... B.......... C.......... D.......... E..........

346. A. T   B. T   C. T   D. T   E. T

The British Thoracic Society recommends that empirical therapy 'should always cover' *Strep. pneumoniae*. The preferred regimen is amoxicillin or penicillin; when *Legionella* or *M. pneumoniae* is specifically suspected, erythromycin should be given; antibiotics directed against *Staph. aureus* should be considered during epidemics of influenza. Nosocomial infection due to *Ps. aeruginosa* is treated with an aminoglycoside and an antipseudomonal β-lactam antibiotic (e.g. ceftazidime or mezlocillin).

347. A. F   B. T   C. F   D. F   E. T

The intensity of wheezing is an unreliable indicator of severity; more reliable indicators include respiratory distress at rest, difficulty in speaking sentences, use of accessory muscles of respiration, tachypnoea and tachycardia. Systemic glucocorticoids speed the resolution of severe exacerbations refractory to bronchodilator therapy and are always used as first-line therapy in the management of severe acute asthma. The β-adrenergic agonists are used as first-line therapy in acute asthma; β-blockers are contraindicated. Although the mechanism of action of theophylline is unclear, its effects are due to bronchodilatation, anti-inflammatory effect, improved contractility of the diaphragm, improved clearance of mucus, improved cardiac output, increased diuresis and decreased vascular permeability. Ipratropium bromide, an anticholinergic agent, is useful in refractory cases.

348. A. F   B. T   C. T   D. T   E. T

Noradrenaline is a potent bronchodilator and in the past was used in the acute management of asthma. β-blockers, aspirin, ACE inhibitors and inhaled pentamidine can cause bronchospasm.

349. *Drugs that decrease theophylline clearance include*

A. phenytoin.
B. phenobarbital.
C. rifampicin.
D. carbamazepine.
E. frusemide.

A............   B..........   C..........   D..........   E..........

350. *Recognised features of chronic obstructive lung disease include the following:*

A. it is unusual in the absence of a history of cigarette smoking.
B. α_1-antitrypsin deficiency is associated with disease that is prominent in the upper lung zones.
C. chest X-ray often shows low flattened diaphragm.
D. when forced expiratory volume in 1 second (FEV_1) falls to less than 1 litre, 5-year survival is approximately 50%.
E. diffusion capacity of carbon monoxide is increased in the presence of emphysema.

A............   B..........   C..........   D..........   E..........

351. *A 65-year-old patient with long-standing chronic obstructive airways disease is admitted to the accident and emergency department. The following statements about management are correct.*

A. Oxygen (90–100%) is usually mandatory.
B. Ipratropium bromide and β-adrenergic agonists are equally effective in the management of bronchospasm.
C. Combination therapy with ipratropium bromide and β-adrenergic effects is more effective than either of these drugs alone.
D. Glucocorticoids should be avoided.
E. In the absence of pneumonia, antibiotics should be avoided.

A............   B..........   C..........   D..........   E..........

352. *Recognised features of cystic fibrosis include the following:*

A. sweat testing for chloride greater than $60\,mEq\,l^{-1}$ remains the gold standard for the diagnosis of cystic fibrosis.
B. the lower lung lobes are generally more involved than the upper lobes.
C. lung function tests are consistent with a restrictive abnormality.
D. *Ps. aeruginosa* is the most characteristic organism cultured in sputum culture.
E. pulmonary disease accounts for most of the morbidity and mortality.

A............   B..........   C..........   D..........   E..........

349. A. F   B. F   C. F   D. F   E. F

All these drugs increase theophylline clearance. Drugs that decrease theophylline clearance include cimetidine, caffeine, calcium channel blockers, propranolol, isoniazid, macrolide antibiotics, quinolone antibiotics including ciprofloxacin, and allopurinol.

350. A. T   B. F   C. T   D. T   E. F

Chronic obstructive lung disease is unusual in the absence of a history of cigarette smoking. α_1-Antitrypsin deficiency should be considered in non-smokers or young patients with emphysema; in these patients the disease tends to show a basilar predominance. The chest X-ray shows low flattened diaphragm in chronic obstructive lung disease and in emphysema there may be bullae, reduced vascular marking and hyperlucent lung fields. FEV_1 allows objective assessment of severity of the disease and is also a prognostic marker: when FEV_1 falls to less than 1 litre, 5-year survival is approximately 50%. In emphysema, the diffusion capacity of carbon dioxide is reduced.

351. A. F   B. T   C. F   D. F   E. F

High-dose oxygen should be avoided because it eliminates the hypoxic drive, exacerbating the hypercapnia. Both β-adrenergic agonists and ipratropium bromide are equally effective in ameliorating bronchospasm but combination therapy has no further effect. Although the role of steroids in the management of acute exacerbations is controversial, they are often used. Antibiotics are useful in those with underlying severe lung disease or more severe exacerbations.

352. A. T   B. F   C. F   D. T   E. T

Sweat testing (by pilocarpine iontophoresis method) for chloride greater than $60\,mEq\,l^{-1}$ remains the gold standard for the diagnosis of cystic fibrosis. Pulmonary disease accounts for most of the morbidity and mortality in cystic fibrosis and chest radiography reveals increased reticular and interstitial marking, bronchiectasis and hilar adenopathy. Generally the upper lobes are more severely involved than the lower lobes. Lung function tests show obstructive pathology including bronchial hyperreactivity and air trapping. In later stages, hypoxaemia and hypercapnia occur. Sputum cultures are mandatory during acute exacerbations and are usually associated with *Ps. aeruginosa*. Other organisms commonly seen are *Staph. aureus*, *Ps. cepacia* and *H. influenzae*.

353. *Extrapulmonary manifestations of cystic fibrosis include*

    A. rectal prolapse.
    B. diabetes mellitus.
    C. biliary cirrhosis.
    D. infertility.
    E. growth retardation.

    A...........   B..........   C..........   D..........   E..........

354. *In a 17-year-old patient with cystic fibrosis the management includes the following:*

    A. intravenous antibiotics are the treatment of choice in acute exacerbations.
    B. bronchodilators are contraindicated.
    C. nebulised recombinant deoxyribonuclease 1 (rhDNase 1).
    D. glucocorticoids are mandatory during acute exacerbations.
    E. lung transplantation is contraindicated in these patients because of poor survival.

    A...........   B..........   C..........   D..........   E..........

355. *Predisposing factors for thromboembolism include*

    A. cardiac failure.
    B. recent pelvic surgery.
    C. prolonged immobilisation.
    D. pregnancy.
    E. menarche.

    A...........   B..........   C..........   D..........   E..........

356. *The diagnosis of pulmonary embolism was made in a 65-year-old patient with dense hemiplegia. Recognised clinical manifestations include*

    A. iliofemoral thrombosis.
    B. pleuritic chest pain.
    C. haemoptysis.
    D. loud pulmonary second heart sound.
    E. tachycardia.

    A...........   B..........   C..........   D..........   E..........

353.   A. T   B. T   C. T   D. T   E. T

Extrapulmonary manifestations of this disease include failure to thrive, growth retardation, meconium ileus, rectal prolapse, biliary cirrhosis, gallstones, intussusception, male infertility, diabetes mellitus and hypertrophic pulmonary osteoarthropathy.

354.   A. T   B. F   C. T   D. F   E. F

The management of cystic fibrosis is directed towards reducing the burden of infection and improving airflow and bronchial hygiene. Intravenous antibiotics are the treatment of choice during an acute exacerbation and usually include a combination of a semi-synthetic penicillin and a third-generation cephalosporin, which are directed against *Ps. aeruginosa* pending the reports of sputum cultures. Aerosolised tobramycin has been shown to reduce the density of *Ps. aeruginosa* and improve lung function in patients with clinically stable cystic fibrosis. Bronchodilators are useful in those with bronchospasm and chest physiotherapy can help in removing mucus. The use of glucocorticoids is controversial in the setting of bacterial infection due to their growth-retardation effects with long-term use. Recombinant deoxyribonuclease improves the consistency of sputum, improves pulmonary function and reduces the need for parenteral antibiotics. Lung transplantation should be considered in those with severe hypoxaemia, hypercapnia; 1-year survival after lung transplantation is about 60%.

355.   A. T   B. T   C. T   D. T   E. F

Predisposing factors for thromboembolism include surgery (particularly of the leg, pelvis, lower abdomen or after prostatectomy), following cerebrovascular accident (about half of the patients develop deep venous thrombosis (DVT)), following myocardial infarction (one-third of patients have DVT), obesity, malignancy, varicose veins, oral contraceptives, older age (exponential increase above the age of 50 years), immobilisation (paralysed limbs in stroke, paraplegia), previous DVT (the risk increases two- to three-fold), pregnancy (increased risk in the postpartum period), tissue trauma and hypercoagulable states (antithrombin III deficiency, protein C deficiency, protein S deficiency, antiphospholipid syndrome, excessive plasminogen activator inhibitor, polycythaemia vera, erythrocytosis).

356.   A. T   B. T   C. T   D. T   E. T

The clinical features of pulmonary embolism depend on the severity of involvement of the pulmonary vasculature and range from non-specific features to tachycardia, tachypnoea and even sudden death. Common presenting features include pleuritic chest pain, cough and apprehension. The presence of haemoptysis indicates that the patient has pulmonary infarction. On examination the patient may be tachypnoeic and have a loud pulmonary second heart sound, inspiratory crackles and pleural rub.

357. *Recognised features of pulmonary embolism on diagnostic studies include the following:*

A. arterial hypercapnia on blood gas analysis.
B. ECG may show left heart strain.
C. the ventilation–perfusion scan (V/Q scan) is most useful when it is concordant with the clinician's pre-test suspicion of pulmonary embolism.
D. pulmonary angiography is mandatory in all patients for diagnosis.
E. evaluation for DVT may support diagnosis, particularly when V/Q scans are non-diagnostic.

A........... B.......... C.......... D.......... E..........

358. *The following statements about the management of pulmonary embolism are correct.*

A. Intravenous anticoagulation should not be started until definitive diagnosis is made.
B. Oral warfarin therapy is overlapped with intravenous heparin therapy.
C. Inferior vena caval interruption is considered in patients with recurrent emboli despite adequate anticoagulation.
D. Thrombolytic therapy should be considered in patients who are haemodynamically unstable following massive acute embolism.
E. Pulmonary embolectomy should be considered in all patients with proven pulmonary emboli.

A........... B.......... C.......... D.......... E..........

359. *Recognised causes of haemoptysis include*

A. mitral stenosis.
B. tuberculosis.
C. pulmonary arteriovenous malformations.
D. mesothelioma.
E. Goodpasture's syndrome.

A........... B.......... C.......... D.......... E..........

357.　A. F　　B. F　　C. T　　D. F　　E. T

Arterial blood gas analysis may show hypoxaemia and hypocapnia, depending on the extent of involvement of the pulmonary circulation. ECG features include sinus tachycardia, right heart strain (P pulmonale, tall QRS complexes in lead V1, S1S2S3 syndrome, S1Q3T3 syndrome), atrial fibrillation or atrial flutter. Chest X-ray findings include normal X-ray, subsegmental atelectasis, pleural effusion, lower lobe infiltrates or hyperlucency of the lung fields due to oligaemia. V/Q scans are mandatory in all patients with suspected pulmonary embolism and are clinically stable. The V/Q scan is most useful when it is concordant with the clinician's pre-test suspicion of pulmonary embolism. Evaluation for DVT may support diagnosis, particularly when V/Q scans are non-diagnostic. Pulmonary angiography is used only when clinical data and non-invasive tests are not diagnostic, particularly when the risks of anticoagulation are high or when thrombolytic therapy or inferior vena caval interruption is considered.

358.　A. F　　B. T　　C. T　　D. T　　E. F

Intravenous anticoagulation should not be withheld for a definitive diagnosis to be made, unless there are absolute contraindications. Oral warfarin therapy is overlapped for 3–5 days with intravenous heparin therapy because of the risk of increased thrombosis in the first few days of oral anticoagulant therapy. Inferior vena caval interruption is considered in patients with recurrent emboli despite adequate anticoagulation (including residual emboli in the legs and patients with compromised cardiopulmonary function who may not withstand a recurrent event), in those in whom anticoagulants are absolutely contraindicated, in those with paradoxical emboli in patent foramen ovale and with septic emboli, and in those undergoing pulmonary embolectomy. Thrombolytic therapy should be considered in patients who are haemodynamically unstable following massive acute embolism. Pulmonary embolectomy is considered only rarely, even in patients with angiographically proven pulmonary emboli who remain in shock despite thrombolytics.

359.　A. T　　B. T　　C. T　　D. F　　E. T

Causes of haemoptysis include bronchial neoplasms (carcinoma, adenoma), lung infection (bronchitis, tuberculosis, pneumonia or lung abscess), mitral stenosis, pulmonary emboli, pulmonary arteriovenous malformations, Goodpasture's syndrome and Wegener's granulomatosis.

360. *The following statements about ARDS are correct.*

   A. The diagnosis requires exclusion of other causes of lung oedema.
   B. Patients have severe hypoxaemia despite high fractional concentration of inspired oxygen.
   C. Large pleural effusions are a common feature.
   D. Positive end-expiratory pressure ventilation is contraindicated.
   E. With adequate treatment mortality remains low.

   A........... B.......... C.......... D.......... E..........

361. *The following statements about pneumonia in immunocompromised hosts are correct.*

   A. Empirical antibiotic therapy should include coverage of *Staph. aureus* and *Ps. aeruginosa.*
   B. Amphotericin should be avoided in those with evidence of superficial fungal infection.
   C. *P. carinii* pneumonia may occur as upper lobe infiltrates in those receiving prophylactic pentamidine therapy.
   D. Glucocorticoid therapy is contraindicated in *P. carinii* pneumonia.
   E. Trimethoprim–sulphamethoxazole therapy is contraindicated in *P. carinii* pneumonia.

   A........... B.......... C.......... D.......... E..........

362. *The following statements about lung abscess are correct.*

   A. Foul-smelling sputum suggests anaerobic bacteria.
   B. Gingival infections are a predisposing factor.
   C. Carcinoma of the lung is a recognised cause.
   D. Intravenous penicillin is adequate for anaerobic infections.
   E. Most patients require surgical resection for complete cure.

   A........... B.......... C.......... D.......... E..........

363. *The following statements about the management of sarcoidosis are correct.*

   A. Most patients with sarcoidosis develop chronic disease with time.
   B. Glucocorticoids are contraindicated in uveitis.
   C. Corticosteroid treatment is usually begun in asymptomatic patients with no evidence of clinical or radiological progression.
   D. Methotrexate is beneficial in steroid-resistant sarcoid disease.
   E. Inhaled glucocorticosteroids are the treatment of choice in sarcoidosis.

   A........... B.......... C.......... D.......... E..........

360. A. T   B. T   C. F   D. F   E. F

ARDS is usually associated with sepsis, major trauma, drug overdose and lung aspiration particularly from the stomach. The diagnosis requires exclusion of other causes of lung oedema. Patients have severe hypoxaemia despite high fractional concentration of inspired oxygen. Large pleural effusions are unusual and indicate a secondary aetiology and chest X-rays usually demonstrate lung infiltrates without pulmonary vascular redistribution. Positive end-expiratory pressure ventilation with haemodynamic monitoring is the treatment of choice to maintain arterial oxygen concentrations. Despite adequate treatment, mortality is as high as 50% and often is due to accompanying failures of other organs.

361. A. T   B. F   C. T   D. F   E. F

In immunocompromised hosts, empirical therapy before microbial tests are available should include broad-spectrum antibiotics; these should cover *Staph. aureus* and *Ps. aeruginosa*. Amphotericin should be included in those with evidence of superficial fungal infection. *P. carinii* pneumonia may occur as upper lobe infiltrates in those receiving prophylactic pentamidine therapy. Glucocorticoid therapy has been shown to be beneficial in moderately severe *P. carinii* pneumonia. The treatment of choice for *P. carinii* pneumonia is trimethoprim–sulphamethoxazole therapy.

362. A. T   B. T   C. T   D. T   E. F

Anaerobic organisms are a common cause of lung abscess and are suggested by foul-smelling sputum. Anaerobic infections usually respond to intravenous penicillin alone, although addition of clindamycin may hasten the process of resolution. Healing may take up to 12–18 months and surgical therapy is rarely required. Other causes of lung abscess include tuberculosis, fungal infections, infections with *Staph. aureus* and Gram-negative bacilli, septic emboli and carcinoma.

363. A. F   B. F   C. F   D. F   E. F

Only one-third of the patients who present with sarcoidosis develop chronic disease; the remainder show complete resolution or improvement in symptoms or radiological abnormalities occurs. Glucocorticoids are useful in uveitis or when there is impairment of vital organs, such as kidney, heart, brain or progressive liver involvement. Steroid therapy is seldom required in asymptomatic patients with no evidence of clinical or radiological progression. Inhaled steroids are of no benefit in sarcoid lung disease. Although methotrexate is useful in the management of mucocutaneous sarcoidosis, it is of no benefit in those with pulmonary involvement.

364. *Recognised causes of obstructive sleep apnoea include*

    A. obesity.
    B. tonsillar hypertrophy.
    C. acromegaly.
    D. hypothyroidism.
    E. nasal obstruction.

    A...........   B..........   C..........   D..........   E..........

365. *A 35-year-old man has obesity, nasal septal deviation and obstructive sleep apnoea. Management of the sleep apnoea includes*

    A. Nasal continuous positive airway pressure (CPAP).
    B. tracheostomy.
    C. weight reduction.
    D. correction of septal deviation.
    E. avoidance of alcohol.

    A...........   B..........   C..........   D..........   E..........

366. *The following statements about lung transplantation are correct.*

    A. Single-lung transplantation is mandatory for bronchiectasis.
    B. Double-lung transplantation is mandatory for cystic fibrosis.
    C. Eisenmenger's syndrome is a contraindication for lung transplantation.
    D. Single-lung transplantation is the procedure of choice for fibrotic restrictive disease.
    E. Lung transplantation is usually most effective in acutely ill patients in respiratory failure.

    A...........   B..........   C..........   D..........   E..........

367. *A 33-year-old man developed acute respiratory symptoms including high fever and cough. Chest X-ray showed consolidation of the right mid-zone. Leucocyte count was $4.0 \times 10^9/l$ with a normal differential count. Attempts to make a blood smear were not successful as the erythrocytes agglutinated. No bacterial pathogens were cultured.*

    A. This patient most probably has *M. pneumoniae* infection.
    B. The agglutination is probably due to the presence of cold haemagglutinins.
    C. The absence of leucocytosis makes *Mycoplasma* infection unlikely.
    D. *M. pneumoniae* infection is rare in winter months.
    E. The treatment is erythromycin.

    A...........   B..........   C..........   D..........   E..........

364.   A. T   B. T   C. T   D. T   E. T

Causes of obstructive sleep apnoea include tonsillar or adenoidal hypertrophy, obesity, nasal obstruction, vocal cord paralysis, micrognathia, bulbar neuro-muscular disease and causes of macroglossia (e.g. acromegaly, hypothyroidism).

365.   A. T   B. T   C. T   D. T   E. T

The management of obstructive sleep apnoea includes management of the underlying cause, e.g. correction of nasal septal deviation, removal of enlarged adenoids and uvulopalatopharyngoplasty. Nasal CPAP is usually the treatment of choice in these patients. Tracheostomy is the most effective treatment but requires special care as it interferes with speech and mucociliary clearance and is thus reserved for disabling hypersomnolence or life-threatening hypoxaemia.

366.   A. F   B. T   C. F   D. T   E. F

Single-lung transplantation is the procedure of choice in fibrotic restrictive lung disease, whereas double-lung transplantation is mandatory for bronchiectasis and cystic fibrosis where there is risk of spillover infection from the native lung. Heart–lung transplantation is indicated in patients with combined lung and heart disease, such as Eisenmenger's syndrome. Lung transplantation is not used in the management of acutely ill patients in respiratory failure.

367.   A. T   B. T   C. F   D. F   E. T

This patient probably has *M. pneumoniae* infection and about half these patients have cold agglutinins. Like all pneumonias it is common in winter months. Absence of leucocytosis is a frequent feature of this infection. The diagnosis is confirmed by a positive complement fixation test and the presence of cold haemagglutinins. Patients respond to erythromycin or tetracycline therapy.

368. *Extrapulmonary manifestations of* Mycoplasma *pneumonia include*

    A. myocarditis.
    B. erythema multiforme.
    C. arthritis.
    D. glomerulonephritis.
    E. autoimmune haemolytic anaemia.

    A...........   B..........   C..........   D..........   E..........

369. *In a 65-year-old patient with wheeze the arterial blood gases analysis showed* P_{O_2} *56 mmHg (7.3 kPa),* P_{CO_2} *75 mmHg (9.8 kPa), bicarbonate 25 mEq l^{-1} and pH 7.2. His blood pressure is 240/110 mmHg.*

    A. This patient has metabolic acidosis.
    B. The patient should be treated with 100% oxygen.
    C. The blood gas picture is most likely due to acute exacerbation of asthma.
    D. His blood pressure should be treated with metoprolol.
    E. Lung function tests will show a restrictive picture.

    A...........   B..........   C..........   D..........   E..........

370. *Causes of dullness at a lung base on percussion include*

    A. emphysema.
    B. pleural effusion.
    C. pleural thickening.
    D. consolidation of the lung.
    E. raised hemidiaphragm.

    A...........   B..........   C..........   D..........   E..........

371. *Causes of an exudative pleural effusion include*

    A. cardiac failure.
    B. nephrotic syndrome.
    C. hypothyroidism.
    D. tuberculosis.
    E. bronchogenic carcinoma.

    A...........   B..........   C..........   D..........   E..........

372. *Recognised causes of bloody pleural fluid include*

    A. malignancy.
    B. pulmonary embolus.
    C. cardiac failure.
    D. tuberculosis.
    E. trauma to the chest.

    A...........   B..........   C..........   D..........   E..........

368. A. T   B. T   C. T   D. T   E. T

Extrapulmonary manifestations of *Mycoplasma* pneumonia include arthralgia, arthritis, autoimmune haemolytic anaemia, pericarditis, myocarditis, hepatitis, glomerulonephritis, erythema multiforme, Stevens–Johnson syndrome and DIC.

369. A. F   B. F   C. F   D. F   E. F

The blood gas picture is most commonly associated with acute exacerbation of chronic bronchitis and the patient has respiratory acidosis. If the arterial Po_2 is less than 8 kPa, administer 24% oxygen. High-dose oxygen will eliminate the hypoxic drive and tends to worsen the condition. β-blockers are contraindicated in patients with severe bronchospasm. Lung function tests should show an obstructive lung picture.

370. A. F   B. T   C. T   D. T   E. T

Causes of dullness at a lung base on percussion include pleural effusion, pleural thickening, consolidation and collapse of the lung and raised hemidiaphragm.

371. A. F   B. F   C. F   D. T   E. T

The protein content of an exudate is more than $3\,g\,l^{-1}$. Causes for an exudate include bronchogenic carcinoma, secondaries in the pleura, pneumonia, pulmonary infarction, tuberculosis, rheumatoid arthritis, systemic lupus erythematosus, lymphoma and mesothelioma. Causes of a transudate include nephrotic syndrome, cardiac failure, liver cell failure and hypothyroidism.

372. A. T   B. T   C. F   D. T   E. T

Haemorrhagic pleural fluid is seen in malignancy, pulmonary embolus, tuberculosis and trauma to the chest.

373. *Indicators of a very severe life-threatening attack of acute asthma include*

A. pulsus paradoxus.
B. hypertension.
C. normal or increased carbon dioxide tension.
D. severe hypoxia.
E. low pH.

A............ B.......... C.......... D.......... E..........

374. *Wheeze is a prominent sign in*

A. acute left ventricular failure.
B. polyarteritis nodosa.
C. eosinophilic lung disease
D. recurrent thromboembolism.
E. pleural effusion.

A............ B.......... C.......... D.......... E..........

375. *Complications of bronchiectasis include*

A. pleural effusion.
B. pneumothorax.
C. brain abscess.
D. amyloidosis.
E. sinusitis.

A............ B.......... C.......... D.......... E..........

376. *Causes of cor pulmonale include*

A. obesity.
B. kyphoscoliosis.
C. high altitude.
D. lung resection.
E. primary pulmonary hypertension.

A............ B.......... C.......... D.......... E..........

377. *The following statements about cystic fibrosis are correct.*

A. An elevated sweat sodium has a greater predictive value for diagnosis in adults compared with children.
B. It can be diagnosed in infancy by the immunoreactive trypsin assay of dried blood.
C. It is due to a defect of the chloride channels at the luminal surface of the airway epithelial cells.
D. Median lifespan is about 60 years.
E. Bilateral lung transplantation should be avoided in these patients.

A............ B.......... C.......... D.......... E..........

373. A. F   B. F   C. T   D. T   E. T

Indicators of a very severe life-threatening attack of acute asthma include normal or increased carbon dioxide tension, severe hypoxia and low pH. Pulsus paradoxus is a poor guide to the severity of acute asthma as it compares poorly with the measurement of peak flow. Hypertension is not an indicator of the severity of asthma.

374. A. T   B. T   C. T   D. T   E. F

Wheeze is a prominent sign in chronic obstructive airway disease, acute left ventricular failure, polyarteritis nodosa, eosinophilic lung disease, recurrent thromboembolism and tumour causing localised wheeze.

375. A. T   B. T   C. T   D. T   E. T

Complications of bronchiectasis include pneumonia, pleurisy, pleural effusion, pneumothorax, sinusitis, haemoptysis, brain abscess and amyloidosis.

376. A. T   B. T   C. T   D. T   E. T

Causes of cor pulmonale include obesity, kyphoscoliosis, high altitude, lung resection, primary pulmonary hypertension, pulmonary emboli, vasculitis of the small pulmonary arteries, chronic obstructive lung disease, chronic persistent asthma and interstitial fibrosis.

377. A. F   B. T   C. T   D. F   E. F

A sweat sodium concentration over $60\,mEq\,l^{-1}$ is indicative of cystic fibrosis. It identifies over 75% by the age of 2 years and about 95% by the age of 12 years. It is more difficult to interpret in older children and adults. Cystic fibrosis can be diagnosed in infancy by the immunoreactive trypsin assay of dried blood. It is due to a defect of the chloride channels at the luminal surface of the airway epithelial cells. The median age of survival is currently in the early thirties. It is estimated that at least half of those with cystic fibrosis will be adults by the year 2000. Bilateral lung transplantation is necessary in this condition to avoid contamination of the donor lung by spillover of infected material from the recipient's remaining lung.

378. *Causes of pneumothorax include*

   A. cystic fibrosis.
   B. Marfan's syndrome.
   C. carcinoma lung.
   D. emphysematous bullae.
   E. bronchial asthma.

   A.......... B.......... C.......... D.......... E..........

379. *Tension pneumothorax should be suspected in the presence of*

   A. hyperthermia.
   B. hypotension.
   C. severely progressive dyspnoea.
   D. severe tachycardia.
   E. marked mediastinal shift.

   A.......... B.......... C.......... D.......... E..........

380. *Causes of lung collapse include*

   A. bronchogenic carcinoma.
   B. mucous plugs of asthma.
   C. Brock's syndrome.
   D. hilar adenopathy.
   E. bronchial adenoma

   A.......... B.......... C.......... D.......... E..........

378. A. T   B. T   C. T   D. T   E. T

Causes of pneumothorax include spontaneous (usually in thin males), trauma, bronchial asthma, chronic obstructive airways disease (emphysematous bullae), carcinoma of the lung, cystic fibrosis, tuberculosis, mechanical ventilation, Marfan's syndrome, Ehlers–Danlos syndrome and catamenial pneumothorax.

379. A. F   B. T   C. T   D. T   E. T

Tension pneumothorax should be suspected in the presence of severe progressive dyspnoea, severe tachycardia, hypotension and marked mediastinal shift.

380. A. T   B. T   C. T   D. T   E. T

Causes of lung collapse include bronchogenic carcinoma, mucous plugs (asthma, allergic bronchopulmonary aspergillosis), extrinsic compression from hilar adenopathy (e.g. primary tuberculosis), tuberculosis (Brock's syndrome) and other intrabronchial tumours including bronchial adenoma.

11 RHEUMATOLOGY AND DISEASES OF BONE

381. *The following statements about bone disease are correct.*

   A. Acute haematogenous osteomyelitis is rarely caused by *Staph. aureus*.
   B. Osteomyelitis in the presence of internal fixation devices cannot usually be eradicated by antimicrobials alone.
   C. *Salmonella* often causes osteomyelitis in haemoglobinopathies.
   D. Osteomyelitis due to diabetes is seldom cured by drug therapy alone.
   E. In chronic myelitis, excision of sequestrum is required for eradication.

   A...........   B..........   C..........   D..........   E..........

382. *The following statements about septic arthritis are correct.*

   A. Non-gonococcal septic arthritis is most often due to *Staph. aureus*.
   B. Non-bacterial septic arthritis usually requires aggressive management including surgical drainage.
   C. It is usually clinically difficult to differentiate septic bursitis of the prepatellar bursa from septic arthritis of the knee.
   D. Surgical drainage should be avoided in septic arthritis of a prosthetic joint.
   E. The antimicrobial coverage for septic arthritis in an immunocompromised patient should include agents active against both staphylococci and Gram-negative bacilli.

   A...........   B..........   C..........   D..........   E..........

383. *Lyme disease*

   A. arthritis usually precedes the annular erythematous skin rash.
   B. is caused by a spirochaete.
   C. is a tick-borne disease
   D. responds to oral doxycycline.
   E. diagnosis is entirely based on serological studies.

   A...........   B..........   C..........   D..........   E..........

381. A. F   B. T   C. T   D. T   E. T

Acute haematogenous osteomyelitis is usually caused by *Staph. aureus.*
Osteomyelitis in the presence of internal fixation devices cannot usually be
eradicated by antimicrobials alone. Removal of foreign material is usually
required for cure. *Staph. aureus* remains the commonest cause of osteomyelitis in
haemoglobinopathies but *Salmonella* is an important causative agent.
Osteomyelitis due to diabetes is seldom cured by drug therapy alone and
patients often require débridement, amputation or revascularisation. In chronic
myelitis, excision of sequestrum (dead and sclerotic bone) is required for
eradication. Long-term antibiotic therapy is used only when surgery is not
feasible.

382. A. T   B. F   C. F   D. F   E. T

Non-gonococcal septic arthritis is most often due to *Staph. aureus*. Non-bacterial
septic arthritis is usually due to viral infections (including hepatitis B, infectious
mononucleosis, mumps, rubella, adenovirus and enterovirus) that are self-
limiting; they tend to resolve with rest and NSAIDs within 6 weeks. Septic
bursitis of the prepatellar bursa can be differentiated from septic arthritis of the
knee by localised superficial swelling, which is fluctuant, and relatively painless
movement of the joint (except for full flexion or extension). Surgical drainage in
septic arthritis is indicated in prosthetic joints. The antimicrobial coverage for
septic arthritis in an immunocompromised patient should include agents active
against both staphylococci and Gram-negative bacilli.

383. A. F   B. T   C. T   D. T   E. F

Lyme disease arthritis is usually preceded by an annular erythematous skin rash
called erythema marginatum chronicum. It is caused by a spirochaete called
Borrelia burgdorferi and is a tick-borne disease. The diagnosis is based on the
clinical picture, including exposure in an endemic area and serology. Serology,
however, often gives false-positive and false-negative results. Lyme disease
responds to oral doxycycline or a combination of probenecid and amoxycillin;
both regimens are usually curative.

384. *The following statements about gout are correct.*

    A. Acute gouty arthritis is usually a polyarticular disease.
    B. Colchicine is most effective if given within the first 12–24 h of an acute attack of gout.
    C. The serum uric acid is normal in about one-third of patients with acute gout.
    D. An elevated uric acid level in an acute attack of gouty arthritis should be aggressively treated to resolve the symptoms.
    E. Allopurinol is used in the management of asymptomatic hyperuricaemia.

    A........... B.......... C.......... D.......... E..........

385. *Risk factors for pseudogout include*

    A. hyperparathyroidism.
    B. haemochromatosis.
    C. hypomagnesaemia.
    D. hypothyroidism.
    E. diabetes mellitus.

    A........... B.......... C.......... D.......... E..........

386. *Recognised features of rheumatoid arthritis include*

    A. symmetric inflammation of synovial tissues.
    B. Felty's syndrome.
    C. Sjögren's syndrome.
    D. vasculitis.
    E. pulmonary fibrosis.

    A........... B.......... C.......... D.......... E..........

387. *The following statements about the management of rheumatoid arthritis are correct.*

    A. If one NSAID is not effective during a 2–3 week trial at full dosage, another should be tried.
    B. Glucocorticoids modify the natural history of rheumatoid arthritis.
    C. Methotrexate retards the progression of bony erosions and cartilage loss.
    D. Gold and pencillamine can be used together.
    E. Synovectomy is usually only of temporary benefit.

    A........... B.......... C.......... D.......... E..........

384.   A. T   B. T   C. T   D. T   E. T

Acute gouty arthritis usually occurs in a single joint of the foot or ankle; occasionally it has a polyarticular onset similar to rheumatoid arthritis. Acute attacks of gouty arthritis usually subside spontaneously over several days and prompt therapy can abort the attack within hours. Drugs used are NSAIDs and colchicine, and steroids when colchicine or NSAIDs are contraindicated. Colchicine is most effective if given within the first 12–24h of an acute attack of gout. The serum uric acid is normal in about one-third of patients with acute gout and should not be manipulated until the acute attack has resolved. Asymptomatic hyperuricaemia is not routinely treated because the risks and cost of therapy outweigh the benefits. Allopurinol, a xanthine oxidase inhibitor, is used to treat hyperuricaemia with recurrent gouty arthritis.

385.   A. T   B. T   C. T   D. T   E. T

Pseudogout is due to the deposition of calcium pyrophosphate crystals in synovial joints, usually the knee. Chondrocalcinosis is seen in about three-quarters of the patients, although its presence is not diagnostic. Risk factors include hyperparathyroidism, haemochromatosis, hypomagnesaemia, diabetes mellitus, hypothyroidism, gout, osteoarthritis and neuropathic joints. NSAIDs are beneficial in the treatment of acute arthritis.

386.   A. T   B. T   C. T   D. T   E. T

Rheumatoid arthritis is a connective tissue disorder with protean manifestations, including characteristic symmetric inflammation of synovial tissues and extra-articular manifestations such as rheumatoid nodules, pulmonary fibrosis, serositis, vasculitis, Felty's syndrome and Sjögren's syndrome. Felty's syndrome includes rheumatoid arthritis, splenomegaly, granulocytopenia, non-healing leg ulcers and recurrent bacterial infections. Sjögren's syndrome is characterised by rheumatoid arthritis, dry mouth, dry eyes, parotid gland enlargement, dental caries and recurrent tracheobronchitis.

387.   A. T   B. F   C. T   D. F   E. T

NSAIDs are used to relieve symptoms and if one NSAID is not effective during a 2–3 week trial at full dosage, another should be tried. Disease-modifying antirheumatic drugs such as pencillamine, gold salts and methotrexate retard the progression of bony erosions and cartilage loss. Glucocorticoids do not modify the natural history of rheumatoid arthritis. As gold and pencillamine have a similar spectrum of toxicity they should not be used together. Synovectomy is usually only of temporary benefit. Total replacement of the joint is usually of long-standing benefit.

388.   *The following statements about spondyloarthropathies are correct.*

A. The sacroiliac joints are characteristically spared in ankylosing spondylitis.
B. The arthritis in Crohn's disease is similar to that of ankylosing spondylitis.
C. High-dose salicylates are usually effective in ankylosing spondylitis.
D. Reiter's syndrome predominantly occurs in young men.
E. About three-quarters of the patients with psoriasis have some form of arthritis.

A.......... B.......... C.......... D.......... E..........

389.   *The following statements about systemic lupus erythematosus are correct.*

A. Antinuclear antibodies are positive in virtually all patients.
B. Antibodies to double-stranded DNA are present in virtually all patients.
C. The presence of antibodies to double-stranded DNA usually correlates with severe or active disease.
D. Serum complement levels often fall during exacerbations of the disease.
E. Serology for syphilis may be positive.

A.......... B.......... C.......... D.......... E..........

390.   *The following statements about drug-induced lupus erythematosus are correct.*

A. Procainamide is responsible for most of the cases.
B. Drugs causing lupus-like syndrome tend to aggravate primary systemic lupus erythematosus.
C. Nephritis is the characteristic feature of drug-induced lupus.
D. Anti-histone antibodies are characteristic of this syndrome.
E. Anti-native DNA antibodies are markedly elevated.

A.......... B.......... C.......... D.......... E..........

388. A. F   B. T   C. F   D. T   E. F

Ankylosing spondylitis is characterised by inflammation and ossification of the joints and ligaments of the spine and sacroiliac joints. Hips and shoulders are the most commonly affected peripheral joints. High-dose salicylates are usually ineffective in controlling pain in ankylosing spondylitis and other NSAIDs, particularly indomethacin, are usually used to alleviate the pain. The arthritis in Crohn's disease or ulcerative colitis has a similar clinical picture as ankylosing spondylitis. Reiter's syndrome predominantly occurs in young men and consists of urethritis, conjunctivitis, oligoarthritis and characteristic skin and mucous membrane involvement. Less than 10% of the patients with psoriasis have arthritis, which manifests as distal interphalangeal joint involvement, symmetrical joint involvement as seen in rheumatoid arthritis, sacroiliitis, asymmetric oligoarticular arthritis and arthritis mutilans.

389. A. T   B. F   C. T   D. T   E. T

Antinuclear antibodies are non-specific but are positive in 95% of patients with systemic lupus erythematosus and it is hard to be certain of the diagnosis in their absence. The positive predictive value of the test increases with higher titres. Antibodies to double-stranded DNA occur in less than half the patients but their presence correlates with severe or active disease, particularly nephritis. Serum complement levels often fall during acute exacerbations and like anti-DNA antibodies are used to monitor the course of the disease. Patients with systemic lupus erythematosus may have false-positive syphilis serology.

390. A. T   B. F   C. F   D. T   E. F

Procainamide is responsible for the majority of the cases; other causes include hydralazine and isoniazid. Drugs causing lupus-like syndrome do not seem to aggravate primary systemic lupus erythematosus. Although multiple organs are affected, nephritis and CNS features are not ordinarily present. Anti-histone antibodies are characteristic of drug-induced lupus, but are not specific for this syndrome; anti-native DNA antibodies are almost never detected. Clinical manifestations and many laboratory features return to normal after the offending drug is withdrawn.

391.   *The following statements about the management of systemic lupus erythematosus are correct.*

A. Minor disease exacerbations such as cytopenia without symptoms should be treated with low dose steroids.
B. Active inflammatory glomerulonephritis should be treated with high-dose prednisolone.
C. Cyclophosphamide should be avoided in lupus nephritis.
D. Renal transplantation should be avoided in renal failure due to systemic lupus erythematosus.
E. Increased incidence of spontaneous abortion is seen in systemic lupus erythematosus.

A........... B.......... C.......... D.......... E..........

392.   *The following associations are correct.*

A. Anti-Smith antibody–systemic lupus erythematosus.
B. Anti-SSA antibody–Sjögren's syndrome.
C. Anti-ribonucleoprotein antibody–mixed connective tissue disease.
D. Anti-centromere antibody–CREST syndrome.
E. Anti-SSB antibody–Sjögren's syndrome.

A........... B.......... C.......... D.......... E..........

393.   *The following associations are correct.*

A. Hypersensitivity vasculitis: medium-sized vessels are involved.
B. Polyarteritis nodosa affects medium-sized vessels in the kidneys.
C. Wegener's granulomatosis affects small-sized vessels in the kidneys.
D. Takayasu's arteritis: small-sized vessels are involved.
E. Giant cell arteritis: small-sized vessels are involved.

A........... B.......... C.......... D.......... E..........

394.   *The following statements about Wegener's granulomatosis are correct.*

A. A positive rheumatoid factor is often seen.
B. It is the same as lymphomatoid granulomatosis.
C. Anti-cytoplasmic antibodies (ANCA) are specific for this condition.
D. All patients have pulmonary involvement.
E. It is caused by the organism *Malassezia furfur.*

A........... B.......... C.......... D.......... E..........

391. A. F   B. T   C. F   D. F   E. T

Serological abnormalities and minor cytopenia unaccompanied by symptoms do not require treatment. Minor systemic symptoms may subside with bed rest. Mild to moderate arthritis, fever and pleuropericarditis subside with NSAIDs or low-dose prednisolone. High-dose prednisolone is used to treat high fever, active inflammatory glomerulonephritis, severe thrombocytopenia, severe haemolytic anaemia and most neurological disturbances. Intravenous administration of bolus doses of methylprednisolone are used to treat rapidly progressive renal disease. Cyclophosphamide is used to treat lupus nephritis with a high histological activity score. Long-term anticoagulation is used in thromboembolism with anti-phospholipid antibody. Renal transplantation is used in patients with systemic lupus erythematosus renal failure and the survival rates of transplantation in these patients is similar to other patients with chronic renal failure. Rarely, there is a recurrence in the transplanted kidney. Pregnancy in systemic lupus erythematosus is associated with an increased incidence of intrauterine death, prematurity and spontaneous abortion.

392. A. T   B. T   C. T   D. T   E. T

Anti-Smith antibody is present in less than one-third of patients with systemic lupus erythematosus but is pathgnomonic of this condition. Anti-SSA or Ro antibody and anti-SSB or La antibody are present in Sjögren's syndrome. Anti-ribonucleoprotein antibody (anti-RNP) occurs in mixed connective tissue disease or overlap syndromes. Anti-centromere antibodies are pathgnomonic of CREST (*c*alcinosis, *R*aynaud's phenomenon, (o)*e*sophageal involvement, *s*clerodactyly and *t*elangiectasia) syndrome.

393. A. F   B. T   C. T   D. F   E. F

Hypersensitivity vasculitis affects small vessels and presents with either rash or nephritis. Polyarteritis nodosa affects medium-sized vessels in kidney, liver, peripheral nerves and gastrointestinal tract; angiography is diagnostic. Wegener's granulomatosis affects small- to medium-sized vessels in the lungs and kidneys. Takayasu's arteritis predominantly affects the aorta. Giant cell arteritis is a granulomatosis arteritis of the aorta and its major branches with a predilection for the extracranial branches of the carotid artery, including the temporal artery.

394. A. T   B. F   C. F   D. F   E. F

Wegener's granulomatosis is an autoimmune disorder with necrotising vasculitis involving the lungs and kidneys, although limited forms of the disease without clinical renal or pulmonary involvement have been described. Positive rheumatoid factor, neutrophilia and ANCA are all non-specific laboratory abnormalities seen in active disease.

395. *Destruction of the tufts of the terminal phalanges is commonly seen in*

    A. gout.
    B. acromegaly.
    C. scleroderma.
    D. secondary hyperparathyroidism.
    E. vinyl chloride disease.

    A........... B.......... C.......... D.......... E..........

396. *Extra-articular manifestations of ankylosing spondylitis include*

    A. apical pulmonary fibrosis.
    B. anterior uveitis.
    C. aortic stenosis.
    D. inflammatory bowel disease.
    E. tricuspid regurgitation.

    A........... B.......... C.......... D.......... E..........

395. A. F   B. F   C. T   D. T   E. T

In gout there are punched-out erosions with overhanging bone around deposits of monosodium urate. In acromegaly there is premature or exaggerated osteoarthritis including osteophyte formation. Destruction of the terminal phalanges is commonly seen in scleroderma, secondary hyperparathyroidism and vinyl chloride disease.

396. A. T   B. T   C. F   D. T   E. F

Ankylosing spondylitis is associated with apical pulmonary fibrosis, anterior uveitis, aortic regurgitation, Achilles tendinitis and inflammatory bowel disease.

12 DERMATOLOGY

397. *Recognised features of vitiligo include the following:*

A. hypomelanosis over bony prominences.
B. white hairs are common in the non–vitiliginous areas.
C. it is associated with autoimmune conditions.
D. there are circulating complement-binding anti-melanocyte antibodies.
E. ultraviolet phototherapyA (PUVA therapy) is contraindicated in vitiligo.

A............ B.......... C.......... D.......... E..........

398. *Vitiligo is associated with*

A. pernicious anaemia.
B. diabetes mellitus.
C. alopecia areata.
D. Graves' disease.
E. Hashimoto's disease.

A............ B.......... C.......... D.......... E..........

399. *The following statements about hyperpigmented conditions are correct.*

A. Freckles are caused by increased melanin production in normal number of melanocytes.
B. Lentigines are caused by an increased number of melanocytes in the basal layer of the epidermis.
C. About 10% of the normal population have isolated *café-au-lait* spots.
D. The pigmentation of Addison's disease is due to increased production of melanocyte-stimulating hormone.
E. The hyperpigmentation of haemochromatosis results from the combination of increased pigment formation in the skin and iron deposition.

A............ B.......... C.......... D.......... E..........

400. *The following associations are correct.*

A. Scleroderma–butterfly rash on the face.
B. Dermatomyositis–Gottron's papules.
C. Dermatomyositis–heliotrope rash on the eyelids.
D. Piebaldism–white forelock of hair.
E. Tuberous sclerosis–hypopigmented ash-leaf macules.

A............ B.......... C.......... D.......... E..........

397. A. T   B. F   C. T   D. T   E. F

Vitiligo consists of circumscribed hypomelanotic macules that progressively
enlarge and which are symmetrically distributed over body orifices and bony
prominences. It runs in families in one-third of cases. White hairs are common
in the hypomelanotic areas. Melanocytes are absent in the macules and in some
patients there are circulating complement-binding anti-melanocyte antibodies.
Vitiligo is associated with autoimmune conditions such as pernicious anaemia,
thyroiditis, hyperthyroidism, myxoedema and diabetes mellitus, but is also found
in healthy individuals. PUVA therapy is useful in some patients but may require
over 200 treatments.

398. A. T   B. T   C. T   D. T   E. T

Vitiligo is associated with organ-specific autoimmune conditions, including
Graves' disease, Hashimoto's disease, pernicious anaemia, diabetes mellitus,
alopecia areata and Addison's disease.

399. A. T   B. T   C. T   D. T   E. T

Freckles are caused by increased melanin production in normal number of
melanocytes. Lentigines are caused by an increased number of melanocytes in
the basal layer of the epidermis. LEOPARD syndrome is an acronym for the
autosomal dominant syndrome with multiple *l*entigines, *e*lectrocardiographic
abnormalities, *o*cular hypertelorism, *p*ulmonary stenosis, *a*bnormal genitalia,
*r*etarded growth and *d*eafness. Peutz–Jeghers syndrome is also dominantly
inherited and consists of numerous lentigines around the mouth, eyes, feet,
hands and eyes in association with gastrointestinal polyps. About 10% of the
normal population have isolated *café-au-lait* spots. *Café-au-lait* spots are a feature
of neurofibromatosis and Albright's syndrome. The pigmentation of Addison's
disease is due to increased production of melanocyte-stimulating hormone. The
hyperpigmentation of haemochromatosis results from the combination of
increased pigment formation in the skin and iron deposition.

400. A. F   B. T   C. T   D. T   E. T

Features of dermatomyositis include flat-topped papules over the neck (Gottron's
papules) and violaceous heliotrope rash on the eyelids. Scleroderma is
characterised by excessive collagen in the dermis.

401. *The following statements are correct.*

A. Busulphan causes Addisonian-like hypermelanosis.
B. Chlorpromazine causes blue-grey pigmentation.
C. Inorganic trivalent arsenicals causes raindrop pigmentation.
D. Addison's disease causes pigmentation of palmar creases.
E. Oral contraceptives cause chloasma.

A........... B.......... C.......... D.......... E..........

402. *The following statements about cutaneous infections are correct.*

A. Erysipelas is almost always caused by group A *Streptococcus*.
B. The cellulitis caused by group A *Streptococcus* is easily distinguishable from that caused by *Staph. aureus* clinically.
C. Lower extremity cellulitis associated with cutaneous ulcers in diabetic patients may be polymicrobial in origin.
D. Meningococcaemia should be considered in any febrile patient with a petechial rash.
E. The rash of Lyme disease is known as erythema marginatum.

A........... B.......... C.......... D.......... E..........

403. *Erythema multiforme is associated with*

A. herpes simplex infection.
B. lymphomas.
C. systemic lupus erythematosus.
D. *Mycoplasma* infection.
E. sulphonamides.

A........... B.......... C.......... D.......... E..........

404. *Recognised manifestations of psoriasis include*

A. erythroderma.
B. Koebner phenomenon.
C. nail pitting.
D. Auspitz sign.
E. Wickham's striae.

A........... B.......... C.......... D.......... E..........

405. *Causes of erythema nodosum include*

A. tuberculosis.
B. β-haemolytic streptococcal infection.
C. oral contraceptives.
D. sarcoidosis.
E. inflammatory bowel disease.

A........... B.......... C.......... D.......... E..........

401. A. T   B. T   C. T   D. T   E. T

Busulphan causes an Addisonian-like hypermelanosis, chlorpromazine causes blue-grey pigmentation, inorganic trivalent arsenicals cause raindrop pigmentation, Addison's disease characteristically causes pigmentation of palmar creases and oral contraceptives cause chloasma.

402. A. T   B. F   C. T   D. T   E. F

Erysipelas is almost always caused by group A *Streptococcus*. The cellulitis caused by group A *Streptococcus* is indistinguishable from that caused by *Staph. aureus* clinically. Lower extremity cellulitis associated with cutaneous ulcers in diabetic patients may be polymicrobial in origin. Meningococcaemia should be considered in any febrile patient with a petechial rash. The rash of Lyme disease is an annular erythematous lesion known as erythema chronicum migrans.

403. A. T   B. T   C. T   D. T   E. T

Erythema multiforme is a self-limiting disorder that affects individuals at any age and is associated with the following conditions: drugs (sulphonamides, salicylates, antimalarials, penicillin, barbiturates, hydantoins); infections (herpes simplex, *Mycoplasma* infection, leprosy, typhoid); malignancy (carcinomas and lymphomas); collagen vascular disease (lupus erythematosus, dermatomyositis, periarteritis nodosa); idiopathic, in 50% of the cases no cause is found.

404. A. T   B. T   C. T   D. T   E. F

Psoriasis frequently affects the skin of the elbows, knees, scalp, intergluteal cleft, lumbosacral regions and the glans penis. Typically the lesions are well demarcated, pink to salmon-coloured plaques covered by silvery-white scales. It can also cause erythroderma, which is scaling and erythema of the whole body. Nail changes occur in about one-third of cases and include pitting, dimpling, onycholysis (separation of the nail plate from the underlying bed), crumbling and thickening. In some patients psoriasis may manifest as pustules or pustular psoriasis. Koebner phenomenon, or the formation of new lesions at the site of trauma, is a recognised manifestation but is not characteristic as it is seen in other conditions such as lichen planus. Auspitz sign is the occurrence of multiple, minute bleeding points when the scale is lifted from the plaque and is characteristic of psoriasis. Wickham's striae are white dots or lines, seen in lichen planus, which are symmetrically distributed particularly about the wrists and elbows and glans penis.

405. A. T   B. T   C. T   D. T   E. T

Erythema nodosum is the most common form of panniculitis and tends to present acutely. Panniculitis is an inflammatory reaction in the subcutaneous tissue that may affect predominantly the connective tissue septa separating lobules of fat or predominantly the lobules of fat themselves. Erythema nodosum is associated with infections (β-haemolytic streptococcal infection, tuberculosis, leprosy), drugs (oral contraceptives), sarcoidosis, inflammatory bowel disease and certain malignancies.

406. *In lichen planus*

   A. the presenting signs are pruritic, purple, polygonal papules.
   B. the lesions resolve spontaneously within a week.
   C. multiple symmetric lesions are characteristic.
   D. mucous membranes are spared.
   E. malar erythema is a prominent feature.

   A........... B.......... C.......... D.......... E..........

407. *In pemphigus vulgaris*

   A. acantholysis is characteristically absent.
   B. the mucosa is spared.
   C. the sera contains IgG antibodies to the intercellular cement substance of skin and mucous membranes.
   D. the bullae are subepidermal.
   E. men are more often affected than women.

   A........... B.......... C.......... D.......... E..........

408. *Bullous pemphigoid*

   A. generally affects elderly individuals.
   B. typically affects flexural areas.
   C. features linear deposits of IgG and C3 in the lamina lucida of the basement membrane.
   D. is a relatively benign condition.
   E. oral involvement usually follows the development of cutaneous lesions.

   A........... B.......... C.......... D.......... E..........

409. *Dermatitis herpetiformis*

   A. is characterised by urticaria.
   B. affects females more often than males.
   C. patients may respond to gluten-free diet.
   D. the skin lesions spare the buttocks.
   E. often develops in the third and fourth decade.

   A........... B.......... C.......... D.......... E..........

410. *Recognised features of Henoch–Schönlein purpura include the following:*

   A. it is a rapidly progressive disorder with a fulminant course.
   B. thrombocytopenia is a characteristic feature.
   C. it is due to circulating IgA-containing immune complexes.
   D. adults are more likely to develop renal involvement.
   E. the presence of IgG indicates a worse prognosis

   A........... B.......... C.......... D.......... E..........

406. A. T   B. F   C. T   D. F   E. F

The presenting signs of lichen planus are pruritic, purple, polygonal, flat-topped papules that may coalesce focally to form plaques. These papules are often highlighted by white dots or lines called Wickham's striae. In over two-thirds of the patients, oral lesions are present as white net-like areas. As in psoriasis, the Koebner phenomenon may be seen in lichen planus. The disorder is self-limiting and usually resolves within 1 or 2 years of onset.

407. A. F   B. F   C. T   D. F   E. F

Pemphigus vulgaris begins in the mouth in over 50% of cases. It is characterised by bullae in the epidermis. Superficial separation of the skin after pressure, trauma or on rubbing the thumb laterally on the surface of the uninvolved skin may cause easy separation of the epidermis (Nikolsky sign). Biopsy shows disruption of epidermal intercellular connections, called acantholysis. The sera contains IgG antibodies to the intercellular cement substance of skin and mucous membranes. Lesional sites show a characteristic net-like pattern of intercellular IgG deposits localised to the sites of developed or incipient acantholysis. The majority of the individuals who develop pemphigus are in the fourth to sixth decades of life; men and women are equally affected.

408. A. T   B. T   C. T   D. T   E. T

Bullous pemphigoid is a relatively benign condition (compared to pemphigus vulgaris) with remissions and exacerbations. Characteristically, tense blisters are present in flexural areas, typically in the elderly. The bullae are subepidermal and immunoelectron microscopy shows linear deposits of IgG and C3 in the lamina lucida of the basement membrane.

409. A. T   B. F   C. T   D. F   E. T

Dermatitis herpetiformis occurs more frequently in males and more often in the third and fourth decade, although it is known to develop at any age after weaning. It is characterised by urticarial plaques and vesicles that are extremely itchy. Characteristically they occur bilaterally and symmetrically, involving the extensor surfaces, elbows, knees, upper back and buttocks. Patients with dermatitis herpetiformis develop antibodies to reticulin and gliadin. Gliadin is a class of protein found in the gluten fraction of flour. Some patients with dermatitis herpetiformis respond to gluten-free diet.

410. A. F   B. F   C. T   D. T   E. T

Henoch–Schönlein or anaphylactoid purpura is a distinct self-limiting vasculitis that occurs in children and young adults. It is a disorder characterised by non-thrombocytopenic purpura, arthralgia, abdominal pain and glomerular nephritis. It is due to circulating IgA-containing immune complexes. It usually lasts between 1 and 6 weeks and subsides without sequelae if renal involvement is mild. The presence of IgG indicates a worse prognosis. Adults are more likely to develop renal involvement.

411. *Recognised causes of telangiectasia include*

A. in outdoor workers in temperate climates.
B. CREST syndrome.
C. dermatomyositis.
D. secondary to irradiation.
E. acne rosacea.

A.......... B.......... C.......... D.......... E..........

412. *Complications of hereditary haemorrhagic telangiectasia include*

A. epistaxis.
B. gastrointestinal haemorrhage.
C. iron-deficiency anaemia.
D. haemoptysis.
E. subarachnoid haemorrhage.

A.......... B.......... C.......... D.......... E..........

413. *Complications of herpes zoster include*

A. corneal ulcerations.
B. meningoencephalitis.
C. Ramsay Hunt syndrome.
D. postherpetic neuralgia.
E. disseminated zoster.

A.......... B.......... C.......... D.......... E..........

414. *Mouth ulcers are seen in*

A. erosive lichen planus.
B. pemphigus vulgaris.
C. Behçet's disease.
D. Stevens–Johnson syndrome.
E. herpes simplex.

A.......... B.......... C.......... D.......... E..........

415. *Causes of hypopigmentation include*

A. haemochromatosis.
B. phenylketonuria.
C. piebaldism.
D. hypopituitarism.
E. albinism.

A.......... B.......... C.......... D.......... E..........

411. A. T   B. T   C. T   D. T   E. T

Telangiectasia is a cluster of dilated capillaries and venules. It is seen on the face in those who work outdoors in temperate or cold climates (e.g. farmers), mitral stenosis, myxoedema and as a transitory phenomenon during pregnancy. It is seen at other sites in scleroderma, secondary to irradiation, dermatomyositis, systemic lupus erythematosus, acne rosacea, lupus pernio, polycythaemia and necrobiosis lipoidica diabeticorum.

412. A. T   B. T   C. T   D. T   E. T

Recognised complications of hereditary haemorrhagic telangiectasia include epistaxis, gastrointestinal haemorrhage, iron-deficiency anaemia, haemoptysis and subarachnoid haemorrhage. Epistaxis usually begins between the ages of 10 and 21; it becomes more severe in later decades in about two-thirds of the affected patients. Gastrointestinal haemorrhage usually does not manifest until the fifth or sixth decade. Arteriovenous malformations, angiodysplasia and telangiectasias are present in the stomach, duodenum, small bowel, colon and liver. Haemoptysis, cyanosis, clubbing, cerebral abscess and embolic stroke are due to pulmonary arteriovenous malformations.

413. A. T   B. T   C. T   D. T   E. T

Complications of herpes zoster include corneal ulcerations, meningoencephalitis, phrenic nerve palsy, gangrene of the affected area, Ramsay Hunt syndrome, postherpetic neuralgia and disseminated zoster including pneumonia. In AIDS patients, varicella zoster may cause multifocal encephalitis, ventriculitis, acute haemorrhagic meningomyeloradiculitis, focal necrotising myelitis and vasculitis of the leptomeningeal arteries.

414. A. T   B. T   C. T   D. T   E. T

Mouth ulcers are seen in erosive lichen planus, pemphigus vulgaris, recurrent aphthous ulcers, Behçet's disease, Stevens–Johnson syndrome and recurrent herpes simplex.

415. A. F   B. T   C. T   D. T   E. T

Hypopigmentation is seen in hypopituitarism, albinism, phenylketonuria, leprosy, burns, radiodermatitis, piebaldism (an autosomal dominant condition manifested by a white forelock) and ash-leaf spots (tuberous sclerosis). In haemochromatosis there is hyperpigmentation.

416. *Raynaud's phenomenon is seen in*

    A. scleroderma.
    B. systemic lupus erythematosus.
    C. dermatomyositis.
    D. rheumatoid arthritis.
    E. mixed connective tissue disorders.

    A........... B.......... C.......... D.......... E..........

417. *Examples of vasospastic conditions include*

    A. carpopedal spasm.
    B. livedo reticularis.
    C. chilblains.
    D. erythromelalgia.
    E. Raynaud's phenomenon.

    A........... B.......... C.......... D.......... E..........

418. *Skin manifestations of systemic lupus erythematosus include*

    A. periungual erythema.
    B. livedo reticularis.
    C. butterfly rash.
    D. Gottron's papules.
    E. alopecia.

    A........... B.......... C.......... D.......... E..........

419. *Livedo reticularis is seen in*

    A. polyarteritis nodosa.
    B. occult malignant neoplasm.
    C. cutaneous marmota.
    D. atherosclerotic microemboli to the skin.
    E. young women.

    A........... B.......... C.......... D.......... E..........

420. *Cutaneous conditions related to heat or cold include*

    A. acanthosis nigricans.
    B. erythema ab igne.
    C. livedo reticularis.
    D. Raynaud's phenomenon.
    E. chilblains.

    A........... B.......... C.......... D.......... E..........

416.   A. T   B. T   C. T   D. T   E. T

Raynaud's phenomenon is associated with a variety of immunological and connective disorders including scleroderma, systemic lupus erythematosus, dermatomyositis, rheumatoid arthritis and mixed connective tissue disorders.

417.   A. F   B. T   C. T   D. T   E. T

Carpopedal spasm is due to tetany and is not a vascular phenomenon. The other four conditions are vasospastic conditions.

418.   A. T   B. T   C. T   D. F   E. T

Skin manifestations of systemic lupus erythematosus include butterfly rash, periungual erythema, nail-fold telangiectasia, alopecia, livedo reticularis, hyperpigmentation, urticaria, purpura and scarring eruption of discoid lupus. Gottron's papules are seen in dermatomyositis.

419.   A. T   B. T   C. F   D. T   E. T

Examples of reticulated rashes include cutaneous marmota and livedo reticularis. Livedo reticularis is seen in systemic lupus erythematosus, polyarteritis nodosa, occult malignant neoplasm, atherosclerotic microemboli to the skin and as physiological phenomenon in young women (it is most apparent on the thighs of young females playing outdoor sports on a cold day).

420.   A. F   B. T   C. T   D. T   E. T

Erythema ab igne is a reticular erythematous or pigmented rash usually on the forelegs (or abdomen) at the site exposed to heat. When present over the anterior abdominal wall or lumbar region (most often due to a hot-water bottle) it indicates that there may an underlying intra-abdominal malignancy. Livedo reticularis, Raynaud's phenomenon and chilblains are all exacerbated by the cold. Acanthosis nigricans has no relation to temperature.

421. *Recognised causes of hirsutism include*

A. Sheehan's syndrome.
B. polycystic ovarian disease.
C. acromegaly.
D. Cushing's syndrome.
E. adrenal tumours.

A........... B.......... C.......... D.......... E..........

422. *Drugs causing increased terminal hair growth include*

A. phenytoin.
B. minoxidil.
C. diazoxide.
D. cyclosporin.
E. androgens.

A........... B.......... C.......... D.......... E..........

423. *Acanthosis nigricans is associated with*

A. diabetes associated with marked insulin resistance.
B. Cushing's syndrome.
C. acromegaly.
D. Stein–Leventhal syndrome.
E. adenocarcinomas.

A........... B.......... C.......... D.......... E..........

424. *Cutaneous manifestations of visceral malignancy include*

A. dermatomyositis.
B. migratory thrombophlebitis.
C. ichthyosis.
D. Paget's disease of the nipple.
E. tylosis.

A........... B.......... C.......... D.......... E..........

425. *Lipoatrophy is associated with*

A. mesangiocapillary glomerulonephritis.
B. localised scleroderma.
C. morphea.
D. chronic relapsing panniculitis.
E. intravenous insulin therapy.

A........... B.......... C.......... D.......... E..........

421.   A. F   B. T   C. T   D. T   E. T

Hirsutism is the male pattern of hair growth in women and consists of excessive terminal hair (androgen-sensitive hair). Polycystic disease or Stein–Leventhal syndrome is the underlying cause in 92% of the women with hirsutism. Cushing's syndrome, adrenal or ovarian tumours, drugs and acromegaly are other causes. Sheehan's syndrome, due to postpartum pituitary necrosis, is associated with hair loss.

422.   A. F   B. F   C. F   D. F   E. T

Phenytoin, minoxidil, diazoxide and cyclosporin cause increase in the growth of vellus hair, whereas androgens increase terminal hair growth.

423.   A. T   B. T   C. T   D. T   E. T

Acanthosis nigricans is velvety black overgrowth of hair seen in the axillae, neck, umbilicus, nipples, groin or facial skin. It is associated with malignant conditions such as adenocarcinomas and lymphomas. It may precede the neoplasm by more than 5 years. In about two-thirds of cases the course parallels that of the tumour, including remission with cure. It is also associated with non-malignant conditions, including Cushing's syndrome, acromegaly and Stein–Leventhal syndrome.

424.   A. T   B. T   C. T   D. T   E. T

Certain skin conditions, including dermatomyositis, migratory thrombophlebitis, ichthyosis, Paget's disease of the nipple and tylosis, are all recognised manifestations of visceral malignancy.

425.   A. T   B. T   C. T   D. T   E. F

Lipoatrophy is associated with subcutaneous administration of insulin, mesangiocapillary glomerulonephritis, localised scleroderma, morphea and chronic relapsing panniculitis.

426. *Cutaneous manifestations of sarcoidosis include*

A. erythema nodosum.
B. micropapular sarcoid.
C. scar infiltration.
D. lupus pernio.
E. rhinophyma.

A............   B...........   C...........   D...........   E...........

427. *Indications for steroids in sarcoidosis include*

A. bilateral hilar adenopathy despite the absence of symptoms.
B. hypercalcaemia.
C. CNS involvement.
D. hepatitis.
E. progressive deterioration in lung function.

A............   B...........   C...........   D...........   E...........

428. *Ocular manifestations of sarcoidosis include*

A. anterior uveitis.
B. retinal neovascularisation.
C. vitreous opacities.
D. choroidal granulomas.
E. optic nerve granulomas.

A............   B...........   C...........   D...........   E...........

429. *Skin lesions usually seen on the shins include*

A. necrobiosis lipoidica diabeticorum.
B. pretibial myxoedema.
C. xanthelasma.
D. erythema ab igne.
E. livedo reticularis.

A............   B...........   C...........   D...........   E...........

430. *The following statements are correct.*

A. Xanthelasmas are due to hypertriglyceridaemia.
B. Eruptive xanthomas are associated with hypertriglyceridaemia.
C. Palmar xanthomas are associated with premature coronary artery disease.
D. Pseudoxanthoma elasticum is due to hypercholesterolaemia.
E. Lipaemia retinalis is associated with chylomicronaemia.

A............   B...........   C...........   D...........   E...........

426.   A. T   B. T   C. T   D. T   E. F

Cutaneous manifestations of sarcoid include erythema nodosum, micropapular sarcoid, scar infiltration, and sarcoid plaques of limbs, shoulders, buttocks and thighs. Rhinophyma is seen in rosacea and is unrelated to sarcoidosis.

427.   A. F   B. T   C. T   D. T   E. T

Specific indications for steroids in sarcoidosis include progressive deterioration in lung function (particularly transfer factor and vital capacity), hypercalcaemia, CNS involvement, hepatitis, severe ocular disease, constitutional symptoms and symptomatic pulmonary lesions.

428.   A. T   B. T   C. T   D. T   E. T

Ocular manifestations of sarcoidosis include anterior uveitis, retinal neovascularisation, vitreous opacities, choroidal granulomas and optic granulomas.

429.   A. T   B. T   C. F   D. T   E. T

Skin lesions usually seen on the shins include erythema nodosum, pretibial myxoedema, diabetic dermopathy, erythema ab igne and livedo reticularis.

430.   A. F   B. T   C. T   D. F   E. T

Xanthelasmas are associated with hypercholesterolaemia but may be present without lipid abnormalities. Eruptive xanthomas are associated with hyper-triglyceridaemia. Palmar xanthomas are associated with premature coronary artery disease. Lipaemia retinalis is associated with chylomicronaemia.

431. *Angioid streaks are seen in*

    A. Paget's disease.
    B. sickle cell disease.
    C. Ehlers–Danlos syndrome.
    D. pituitary disorders.
    E. trauma.

    A.......... B.......... C.......... D.......... E..........

432. *Cardiovascular manifestations of pseudoxanthoma elasticum include*

    A. mitral valve prolapse.
    B. restrictive cardiomyopathy.
    C. renovascular hypertension.
    D. premature coronary artery disease.
    E. peripheral vascular disease.

    A.......... B.......... C.......... D.......... E..........

433. *Hairy leucoplakia*

    A. is commonly seen in non-HIV immunosuppressed patients.
    B. is caused by Epstein–Barr virus.
    C. in seropositive patients is usually a harbinger of rapid progression in AIDS.
    D. should be aggressively treated.
    E. responds to antifungal therapy.

    A.......... B.......... C.......... D.......... E..........

434. *The following statements about Kaposi's sarcoma are correct.*

    A. Classic Kaposi's sarcoma may be present for decades.
    B. About one-third of patients with AIDS-associated Kaposi's sarcoma develop a second malignancy.
    C. The African variety of Kaposi's sarcoma is a benign condition.
    D. Transplantation-associated Kaposi's sarcoma often regresses when immunosuppressive therapy is stopped.
    E. A herpes-like virus has been implicated in the aetiology of Kaposi's sarcoma.

    A.......... B.......... C.......... D.......... E..........

435. *Recognised features of Peutz–Jeghers syndrome include*

    A. pigmented freckles around the lips.
    B. intestinal intussusception.
    C. gastrointestinal haemorrhage.
    D. autosomal dominant inheritance.
    E. intestinal polyps.

    A.......... B.......... C.......... D.......... E..........

431. A. T   B. T   C. T   D. T   E. T

Angioid streaks are seen on fundoscopy and are caused by abnormal elastic tissue in Bruch's membrane of the retina. They are seen in pseudoxanthoma elasticum, Paget's disease, sickle cell disease, Ehlers–Danlos syndrome, pituitary disorders and trauma.

432. A. T   B. T   C. T   D. T   E. T

Cardiovascular manifestations of pseudoxanthoma elasticum include mitral valve prolapse, restrictive cardiomyopathy, renovascular hypertension, premature coronary artery disease and peripheral vascular disease.

433. A. F   B. T   C. T   D. F   E. F

Hairy leucoplakia are whitish hairy lesions on the lateral edges of the tongue caused by Epstein–Barr virus. It may be difficult to distinguish from oral candidiasis, but in contrast it does not rub off or respond to antifungal therapy and may change its appearance daily. In seropositive patients, it is usually a harbinger of rapid progression in AIDS. It seldom requires treatment but if necessary can be treated with ganciclovir or acyclovir.

434. A. T   B. T   C. F   D. T   E. T

Classic Kaposi's sarcoma was initially described in Jews and is found on the legs of elderly men. It is confined to the skin and has an indolent course (may present for many decades) and is not fatal. AIDS-associated Kaposi's sarcoma is found in approximately one-third of patients with AIDS and is more common in homosexuals. About one-third of patients with AIDS-associated Kaposi's sarcoma develop a second malignancy. The African variety is an aggressive invasive tumour that is ultimately fatal. It occurs in children and younger men. Transplantation-associated Kaposi's sarcoma is seen in patients on high-dose immunosuppressive therapy; it often regresses when immunosuppressive therapy is stopped.

435. A. T   B. T   C. T   D. T   E. T

Pigmented freckles around the mouth and intestinal polyps are characteristic features of Peutz–Jeghers syndrome. The polyps are distributed in the following frequencies: small bowel (100%), stomach (25%) and colon (30%). The patient complains of pain in the abdomen due to intestinal intussusception and may have a history of gastrointestinal haemorrhage in the upper gastrointestinal tract and rectal bleeding. The inheritance is autosomal dominant.

436. *Recognised causes of pyoderma gangrenosum include*

 A. ulcerative colitis.
 B. rheumatoid arthritis.
 C. chronic myeloid leukaemia.
 D. multiple myeloma.
 E. chronic active hepatitis.

 A.......... B.......... C.......... D.......... E..........

437. *Recognised features of Sturge–Weber syndrome include*

 A. autosomal dominant inheritance.
 B. port-wine stain in the distribution of the first and second division of the trigeminal nerve.
 C. choroidal haemangiomas on fundal examination.
 D. intracranial 'tramline' calcification on the skull radiograph.
 E. haemangiomas of the iris.

 A.......... B.......... C.......... D.......... E..........

438. *Recognised causes of acne vulgaris include*

 A. occupational exposure to oils.
 B. tetracycline.
 C. steroids.
 D. isoniazid.
 E. retinoic acid.

 A.......... B.......... C.......... D.......... E..........

439. *Alopecia areata is associated with*

 A. Down's syndrome.
 B. vitiligo.
 C. hypogammaglobulinaemia.
 D. Addison's disease.
 E. thyrotoxicosis.

 A.......... B.......... C.......... D.......... E..........

440. *Drugs causing alopecia include*

 A. heparin.
 B. vitamin A.
 C. anticancer drugs.
 D. retinoids.
 E. antithyroid drugs.

 A.......... B.......... C.......... D.......... E..........

436.   A. T   B. T   C. T   D. T   E. T

Pyoderma gangrenosum are necrotic ulcers with purplish overhanging edges, usually seen on the limbs and trunk. Recognised causes include ulcerative colitis, Crohn's disease, chronic active hepatitis, rheumatoid arthritis, chronic myeloid leukaemia, polycythaemia rubra vera, multiple myeloma and IgA monoclonal gammopathy. These lesions are treated with high-dose systemic steroids or intralesional steroids and some regress with treatment of the underlying cause.

437.   A. F   B. T   C. T   D. T   E. T

Sturge–Weber syndrome is the only syndrome of the phacomatoses that does not have a hereditary tendency. It occurs sporadically and has no sexual predilection. Other features include port-wine stain in the distribution of the first and second division of the trigeminal nerve, choroidal haemangiomata on fundal examination, haemangiomas of the episclera and iris, and intracranial 'tramline' calcification on the skull radiograph. Neurological manifestations include Jacksonian epilepsy, contralateral hemianopia, hemisensory disturbance, hemiparesis and hemianopia, and low IQ. The ocular manifestations include choroidal angioma, glaucoma, buphthalmos and optic atrophy.

438.   A. T   B. F   C. T   D. T   E. F

Causes of acne vulgaris include occupational exposure to oils, steroids and isoniazid, whereas tetacyclines and retinoic acid are used in the treatment of acne vulgaris.

439.   A. T   B. T   C. T   D. T   E. T

Alopecia areata is associated with autoimmune conditions (including vitiligo, thyrotoxicosis, Addison's disease and pernicious anaemia), Down's syndrome and hypogammaglobulinaemia.

440.   A. T   B. T   C. T   D. T   E. T

Drugs causing alopecia include heparin, vitamin A, anticancer drugs, retinoids, antithyroid drugs and oral contraceptives.

441. *Causes of leg ulcers include*

    A. leprosy.
    B. vasculitis.
    C. sickle cell anaemia.
    D. varicose veins.
    E. diabetes mellitus.

    A.......... B.......... C.......... D.......... E..........

442. *The following associations regarding nail changes and their aetiology are correct.*

    A. Koilonychia–polycythaemia.
    B. Paronychia–iron-deficiency anaemia.
    C. Nail pitting–alopecia areata.
    D. Nail-fold telangiectasia–dermatomyositis.
    E. Subungual angiofibromas–tuberous sclerosis.

    A.......... B.......... C.......... D.......... E..........

443. *When the environmental temperature is greater than body temperature, heat is lost from the body by*

    A. radiation.
    B. conduction.
    C. convection.
    D. forced convection.
    E. evaporation.

    A.......... B.......... C.......... D.......... E..........

444. *When the core temperature of the body falls below the hypothalamic set-point temperature, the following occur:*

    A. dilatation of cutaneous blood vessels.
    B. the person feels hot.
    C. heat production falls.
    D. the basal metabolic rate falls.
    E. the hypothalamus resets the set point within minutes.

    A.......... B.......... C.......... D.......... E..........

445. *The following statements about the hair follicle are correct.*

    A. The anagen phase is the growth phase.
    B. The telogen phase is the resting phase.
    C. Hair found on the pillow and hairbrush is anagen hair.
    D. Telogen hair can be obtained by traction.
    E. About 90% of the hair of the human scalp is in telogen phase.

    A.......... B.......... C.......... D.......... E..........

441. A. T   B. T   C. T   D. T   E. T

Causes of leg ulcers include venous disorders (varicose veins), diabetes mellitus, leprosy, vasculitis (rheumatoid arthritis, systemic lupus erthematosus, pyoderma gangrenosum), haematological disorders (sickle cell anaemia, spherocytosis), neoplastic disorders (basal cell carcinoma, Kaposi's sarcoma), after cellulitis and fungal infections.

442. A. F   B. F   C. T   D. T   E. T

Koilonychia is seen in iron-deficiency anaemia and thyrotoxicosis. Paronychia is due to nail-fold inflammation and is usually due to infection. Nail pitting is seen in psoriasis and alopecia areata. Telangiectasia is seen in dermatomyositis, scleroderma and collagen vascular disease. Plummer's nails are due to onycholysis and occur in hyperthyroidism, typically on the fourth finger.

443. A. F   B. F   C. F   D. F   E. T

The only mechanism by which heat is lost from the body when environmental temperature is greater than body temperature is by evaporation of sweat, which will occur as long as the relative humidity is less than 100%. For each gram of water that evaporates from the body surface about 575 calories (2.4 lkJ) of heat are lost from the body.

444. A. F   B. F   C. F   D. F   E. F

When the core body temperature falls below hypothalamic set point, compensatory mechanisms include cutaneous vasoconstriction, increase in metabolic rate and shivering. All these will allow the body to return to hypothalamic set-point temperature.

445. A. T   B. T   C. F   D. F   E. F

Each hair follicle has cyclical growth controlled by a constitutional time clock. The cycle has three phases of growth (anagen), a short involutional phase (catagen) and a resting (telogen) phase. The anagen phase lasts 3–5 years and the telogen phase 2–4 years. Hair found on the pillow and hairbrush is telogen hair and can be recognised by the fact that the club is depigmented as well as expanded, whereas an anagen hair obtained by traction is fully melanised. About 70–100 hairs per day are lost from the scalp of a normal person. The human scalp contains about 100 000 follicles and 5–10% are in telogen at any time.

13   MISCELLANEOUS

446. *The following statements are correct.*

   A. Benzathine penicillin G is administered subcutaneously.
   B. Oral nitroglycerin requires the 'first-pass' effect to be activated.
   C. The bioavailability of a drug is the fraction of the total drug dose that ultimately reaches the systemic circulation from the site of administration.
   D. The volume of distribution is a term used to relate the amount of drug in the body to the concentration of drug in plasma.
   E. For the vast majority of drugs, the rates of hepatic and renal elimination are proportional to the plasma concentration of the drug.

   A.......... B.......... C.......... D.......... E..........

447. *Drug clearance is affected by several factors including*

   A. drug distribution throughout the body
   B. blood flow through the organ of clearance.
   C. protein binding to the drug.
   D. activity of the clearance processes in the organs of elimination.
   E. drug concentration in the extracellular compartment.

   A.......... B.......... C.......... D.......... E..........

448. *Drugs that are almost entirely cleared by the kidney include*

   A. aspirin.
   B. carbamazepine.
   C. phenytoin.
   D. gentamicin.
   E. amikacin.

   A.......... B.......... C.......... D.......... E..........

449. *A loading dose is often used for the following drugs:*

   A. digitalis.
   B. aminophylline.
   C. intravenous phenytoin.
   D. aspirin.
   E. ibuprofen.

   A.......... B.......... C.......... D.......... E..........

446.   A. F   B. F   C. T   D. T   E. T

Benzathine penicillin G is a depot preparation administered by deep intramuscular injection; it is very painful when administered subcutaneously. Oral nitroglycerin is metabolised by the liver prior to reaching the systemic circulation; this is known as the first-pass effect. However, it can achieve adequate systemic levels when administered sublingually or transdermally. The bioavailability of a drug is the fraction of the total drug dose that ultimately reaches the systemic circulation from the site of administration. This is calculated by dividing the amount of the drug dose that reaches the circulation from the administration site by the amount of the drug dose that would enter the systemic circulation following direct intravenous injection into the circulation. The bioavailability of a drug in different formulations may change because the overall absorption may differ. This has become a recent concern with the increasing use of generic preparations. The volume of distribution is a term used to relate the amount of drug in the body to the concentration of drug in plasma; this is useful in calculating the loading dose and in appreciating how various changes can affect the drug's half-life. For the vast majority of drugs, the rates of hepatic and renal elimination are proportional to the plasma concentration of the drug. This relationship is often described as the 'first-order' process.

447.   A. F   B. T   C. T   D. T   E. F

Drug clearance is not affected by distribution of the drug throughout the body because clearance mechanisms can act only on drug in the circulation. It is affected by several factors, including blood flow through the organ of clearance, protein binding to the drug and activity of clearance processes in the organs of elimination (e.g. enzyme activity in the liver, glomerular filtration rate and tubular secretion in the kidney).

448.   A. F   B. F   C. F   D. T   E. T

Less than 5% of drugs such as aspirin, carbamazepine and phenytoin are cleared by the kidneys, whereas antibiotics such as tobramycin, amikacin and gentamicin are almost entirely cleared by the kidneys. The dosages for the latter drugs will have to be titrated in renal failure.

449.   A. T   B. T   C. F   D. F   E. F

A loading dose is used to obtain the desired therapeutic concentration rapidly. In determining the amount of drug to be given, one needs to consider the volume of distribution of the drug. The entire loading dose of aminophylline is given intravenously over 20 min rather than rapidly, in order to avoid an initial peak concentration and its resulting toxicity. In the case of phenytoin the loading dose is administered orally due to slower absorption. Administering a standard loading dose (420 mg in a 70-kg man) of phenytoin by the intravenous route carries the risk of cardiac arrest and death. Administration of aspirin and ibuprofen do not require a rapidly attained therapeutic concentration and hence do not require a loading dose.

450. *The following statements about drugs that inhibit absorption of other drugs in the intestine are correct.*

   A. Cholestyramine interacts with digoxin.
   B. Aluminium-containing antacids interact with tetracycline.
   C. Kaolin–pectin suspensions interact with digoxin.
   D. Cimetidine interacts with ketoconazole.
   E. Belladonna alkaloids interact with levodopa.

   A........... B.......... C.......... D.......... E..........

451. *The following statements are correct.*

   A. With each change in drug dose or rate of infusion, a change in steady state occurs.
   B. Steady state is the point when the amount of drug being administered equals the amount being eliminated so that plasma and tissue levels remain constant.
   C. The effects of dose adjustments for drugs with longer half-lives are delayed, the time varying with the drug's half-life.
   D. Three to five half-lives determine the time it takes a drug to reach steady state during accumulation.
   E. When administered intermittently, a drug approaches steady-state concentration over time with a pattern similar to that observed with continuous infusion.

   A........... B.......... C.......... D.......... E..........

452. *The following statements are correct.*

   A. For gentamicin, a trough level obtained immediately before administering the next dose is very useful for making decisions regarding dose adjustments.
   B. For drugs that are administered by infusion or intermittently at short intervals, the best time to draw blood is during steady state.
   C. The therapeutic response of digoxin at a certain plasma level can alter with changes in plasma electrolyte concentration.
   D. Theophylline is metabolised predominantly by the kidney.
   E. In renal failure it is not necessary to adjust the dosing regimen of digoxin.

   A........... B.......... C.......... D.......... E..........

232 500 MCQS FOR MRCP PART 1

450. A. T   B. T   C. T   D. T   E. T

Cholestyramine and colestipol are resins that act by binding bile acids and are used to lower cholesterol. They can also bind to other drugs, such as digoxin and warfarin, and retard their absorption; hence it is generally recommended that other drugs are not ingested within 2 h of administration of cholestyramine or colestipol. Antacids containing metals, such as aluminium, magnesium and calcium or iron salts can form insoluble complexes with tetracycline, which then act as chelating agents. Kaolin–pectin suspensions used for diarrhoea can inhibit the absorption of digoxin. H_2-receptor blockers such as cimetidine elevate gastric pH and thus inhibit the dissolution and consequently the absorption of weak bases such as ketoconazole. Inhibition of gastric emptying by belladonna alkaloids results in increasing degradation of acid-labile drugs such as levodopa.

451. A. T   B. T   C. T   D. T   E. T

Steady state is the point when the amount of drug being administered equals the amount being eliminated so that plasma and tissue levels remain constant. With each change in drug dose or rate of infusion, a change in steady state occurs. Three to five half-lives determine the time it takes a drug to reach steady state during accumulation. When administered intermittently, a drug approaches steady-state concentration over time with a pattern similar to that observed with continuous infusion. The effects of dose adjustments for drugs with longer half-lives are delayed, with the time varying with the drug's half life.

452. A. T   B. T   C. T   D. F   E. F

For many drugs administered intermittently, including gentamicin, a trough level obtained immediately before administering the next dose is very useful for making decisions regarding dose adjustments. For drugs that are administered by infusion or intermittently at short intervals, the best time to draw blood is during steady state. The usefulness of a drug assay is limited by physiological changes that may alter the response at a particular drug concentration. An example of this pharmacodynamic change is the response produced at a certain digoxin level in the presence of altered electrolyte concentration (e.g. potassium, magnesium or calcium). Theophylline is predominantly metabolised by the liver and cigarette smoking can increase its metabolism by inducing the activity of the mixed-function oxidase (P450) system. Digoxin is predominantly excreted by the kidneys and since it has a long half-life and small therapeutic index it is critical that the dosage regimen is adjusted in renal failure.

453. *The followings statements about drug interactions are correct.*

A. Anticholinergics can increase the absorption of digoxin.
B. Metoclopramide can increase the absorption of acid-unstable drugs.
C. Sulphonamides can displace barbiturates bound to serum albumin.
D. Allopurinol can inhibit the metabolism of 6-mercaptopurine.
E. In asthma, when aminophylline is used in combination with aerosolized beta-agonists, it has increased toxicity without additive benefit.

A........... B.......... C.......... D.......... E..........

454. *Cimetidine can inhibit the metabolism of*

A. diazepam.
B. imipramine.
C. lidocaine.
D. propranolol.
E. theophylline.

A........... B.......... C.......... D.......... E..........

455. *Amiodarone inhibits the metabolism of*

A. calcium channel blockers.
B. flecainide.
C. phenytoin.
D. quinidine.
E. β-blockers.

A........... B.......... C.......... D.......... E..........

456. *The metabolism of warfarin is inhibited by*

A. alcohol.
B. metronidazole.
C. phenylbutazone.
D. trimethoprim–Sulphamethoxazole.
E. allopurinol.

A........... B.......... C.......... D.......... E..........

457. *The metabolism of phenytoin is inhibited by*

A. chloramphenicol.
B. clofibrate.
C. isoniazid.
D. valproic acid.
E. phenylbutazone.

A........... B.......... C.......... D.......... E..........

453. A. T   B. T   C. T   D. T   E. T

Anticholinergics which decrease intestinal motility may increase the absorption of drugs, such as digoxin, that are relatively poorly absorbed. Metoclopramide by inhibiting gastric emptying can increase the absorption of acid-unstable drugs. Sulphonamides can displace barbiturates bound to serum albumin, leading to increased levels of free barbiturates with possible toxicity. Allopurinol can inhibit the metabolism of 6-mercaptopurine, the latter having a low therapeutic index; this interaction may result in a potentially life-threatening toxicity. In asthma, when aminophylline is used in combination with aerosolized beta-agonists, it has increased toxicity without additive benefit.

454. A. T   B. T   C. T   D. T   E. T

Cimetidine can inhibit the metabolism of diazepam, imipramine, lidocaine, propranolol, theophylline, quinidine and warfarin.

455. A. T   B. T   C. T   D. T   E. F

Amiodarone inhibits the metabolism of calcium channel blockers, flecainide, phenytoin, quinidine and warfarin. It is important to remember that the half-life of amiodarone is 1–2 months, so that it continues to inhibit drug metabolism for several months after being discontinued.

456. A. T   B. T   C. T   D. T   E. T

The metabolism of warfarin is inhibited by cimetidine, amiodarone, alcohol, metronidazole, phenylbutazone, allopurinol and trimethoprim–sulphamethoxazole.

457. A. T   B. T   C. T   D. T   E. T

The metabolism of phenytoin is inhibited by chloramphenicol, clofibrate, isoniazid, valproic acid, phenylbutazone, disulfiram and dicoumarol.

458. *The following drugs can induce haemolysis in patients with G6PD deficiency:*

    A. aspirin.
    B. nitrofurantoin.
    C. primaquine.
    D. sulphonamides.
    E. vitamin K.

    A........... B.......... C.......... D.......... E..........

459. *In patients with methaemoglobin reductase deficiency, methaemoglobinaemia can be induced by the following drugs:*

    A. nitrites.
    B. sulphonamides.
    C. sulphones.
    D. cisplatin.
    E. propranolol.

    A........... B.......... C.......... D.......... E..........

460. *The following associations are correct.*

    A. Catechol *O*-methyltransferase–sulphamethazine.
    B. Catechol *O*-methyltransferase–L-dopa.
    C. *N*-Acetyltransferase–isoniazid.
    D. Cytochrome P450–diazepam.
    E. *N*-Acetyltransferase–hydralazine.

    A........... B.......... C.......... D.......... E..........

461. *A 30-year-old diabetic woman with ischaemic heart disease, diabetes, chronic psychotic disorder and urinary tract infection had liver function tests that showed a cholestatic picture. Drugs that could have contributed to cholestatic liver disease include:*

    A. aspirin.
    B. sulphonylureas.
    C. erythromycin estolate.
    D. chlorpromazine.
    E. nitrofurantoin.

    A........... B.......... C.......... D.......... E..........

462. *A 40-year-old man with ankylosing spondylitis, diabetic nephropathy and schizophrenia has a neutrophil count less than $500/mm^3$ due to the following:*

    A. captopril.
    B. propranolol.
    C. chlorpropamide.
    D. chlorpromazine.
    E. phenylbutazone.

    A........... B.......... C.......... D.......... E..........

458. A. T   B. T   C. T   D. T   E. T

Drugs commonly leading to haemolysis in G6PD deficiency include 1) Antimalarials (primaquine pamaquine), 2) Sulphonamides and sulphones 3) Analgesics (aspirin, phenacetin), 3) Antibacterials (nitrofurantoins, chloramphenicol, nalidixic acid) 4) Antihelminthics (niridazole, stibophen, β-napthol) and 5) Miscellaneous (Vitamin K analogues, probenecid, methylene blue, dimercaprol).

459. A. T   B. T   C. T   D. T   E. T

Nitrites, sulphonamides and sulphones can induce methaemoglobinaemia in patients with methaemoglobin reductase deficiency.

460. A. F   B. T   C. T   D. T   E. T

Catechol O-methyltransferase is involved in the methylconjugation of L-dopa and methyldopa, whereas N-acetyltransferase is involved in the acetylation of sulphamethazine, sulphadiazine, isoniazid, hydralazine, phenelzine, sulphasalazine, aminosalicylic acid and sulphapyridine. Cytochrome P450 IIC is involved in the metabolism of mephenytoin, mephobarbital, hexobarbital, diazepam and omeprazole. Substrates for cytochrome P450 IID6 include antidepressants, antiarrhythmics, β-blockers, codeine, dextromethorphan and neuroleptics.

461. A. F   B. T   C. T   D. T   E. T

Drugs implicated in cholestatic jaundice include the estolate ester of erythromycin, sulphonylureas, phenothiazines, imipramine, sulphamethoxazole, nitrofurantoin and troleandomycin. Aspirin has been implicated in hepatocellular damage; particularly in children it causes Reye's syndrome.

462. A. T   B. T   C. T   D. T   E. T

Drugs that cause granulocytopenia include captopril, cephalosporins, chlorpropamide, phenothiazines, phenylbutazone, propranolol, tolbutamide, phenytoin and semi-synthetic penicillins.

463. *Recognised causes of fixed drug eruptions include*

A. ibuprofen.
B. sulphonamides.
C. phenolphthalein.
D. dapsone.
E. streptomycin.

A........... B.......... C.......... D.......... E..........

464. *The following statements about benzodiazepines are correct.*

A. Diazepam is contraindicated in status epilepticus.
B. Skeletal muscle spasm is relieved by benzodiazepines.
C. Respiratory depression can occur with oral doses in patients with respiratory compromise.
D. Benzodiazepine dependence may develop after only 4 weeks of therapy.
E. Benzodiazepine toxicity can be increased by concomitant use of cimetidine.

A........... B.......... C.......... D.......... E..........

465. *The following statements about phenothiazines are correct.*

A. Prochlorperazine is useful in the treatment of nausea and vomiting.
B. Intractable hiccups are a contraindication for chlorpromazine.
C. Haloperidol is the drug of choice in the management of agitation and psychosis.
D. Phenothiazines are contraindicated in sundown syndrome.
E. Phenothiazines are contraindicated in dementias with psychotic manifestations.

A........... B.......... C.......... D.......... E..........

466. *Glucocorticosteroids*

A. cause neutropenia.
B. decrease the ability of neutrophils to migrate to extravascular sites.
C. cause eosinophilia.
D. increase serum complement levels.
E. promote cytotoxic activity of natural killer cells.

A........... B.......... C.......... D.......... E..........

238 MCQS FOR MRCP PART 1

463. A. T   B. T   C. T   D. T   E. T

Several drugs have been implicated in fixed drug eruptions, including ibuprofen, sulphonamides, phenolphthalein, dapsone, streptomycin, quinine, gold salts, saccharin, tetracyclines, quinines, aspirin, paracetomol, iodides and hydralazine.

464. A. F   B. T   C. T   D. T   E. T

Emergency management of status epilepticus includes diazepam, which is administered intravenously to abort prolonged seizure episodes. Extreme caution should be used in order to avoid cardiac or respiratory compromise. Respiratory depression can occur with oral doses in patients with respiratory compromise. Skeletal muscle spasm is relieved by benzodiazepines and may be used for brief periods for this purpose. Benzodiazepine toxicity can be increased by concomitant use of cimetidine, alcohol or other CNS depressants. Benzodiazepine dependence may develop after only 4 weeks of therapy. The withdrawal syndrome begins 1–10 days after abrupt cessation of therapy and may last for several weeks.

465. A. T   B. F   C. T   D. F   E. F

Prochlorperazine is useful in the treatment of nausea and vomiting. Intractable hiccups may be controlled with chlorpromazine. Phenothiazines are useful in the treatment of schizophrenia, mania, psychotic depression and dementias with psychotic manifestations. Haloperidol is the drug of choice in the management of agitation and psychosis in patients with delirium or dementia. Sundown syndrome is the appearance of worsening confusion in the evening and is seen in patients with dementia and delirium and in those in unfamiliar environments. Short-term phenothiazine therapy may be useful in the sundown syndrome.

466. A. F   B. T   C. T   D. F   E. F

Glucocorticosteroids cause a transient elevation of neutrophils due to an increase in half-life, increased bone marrow release and decreased egress from the circulation to extravascular sites of inflammation. Glucocorticosteroids also cause monocytopenia, lymphocytopenia (selective depletion of $CD4^+$ T cells), eosinopenia and basophilopenia. They have little effect on the function of neutrophils and natural killer cells but profoundly alter the function of eosinophils and T and B lymphocytes. They have little effect on complement but decrease the production of other soluble mediators, including prostaglandins, histamine, leukotrienes, interleukin-1, interleukin-2, interferon γ and tumour necrosis factor α, and decrease the clearance of antigen–antibody complexes from the circulation.

467. *Recognised complications of glucocorticosteroid therapy include*

A. insomnia.
B. acne vulgaris.
C. pseudotumour cerebri.
D. pancreatitis.
E. osteoporosis.

A............ B.......... C.......... D.......... E..........

468. *Indications for pulse regimens for steroids include*

A. recrudescence of disease despite steroid therapy.
B. flare of disease activity in patients who have steroid side-effects.
C. the need to control disease until another treatment modality becomes effective.
D. the onset of rapidly progressive steroid-responsive syndrome.
E. over activity of the hypothalamic–pituitary axis.

A............ B.......... C.......... D.......... E..........

469. *Alterations in drug dosages in the elderly are due to the following changes associated with advancing age:*

A. increase in glomerular filtration rate.
B. increase in hepatic blood flow.
C. altered hepatic conjugation.
D. decline in hepatic oxidative processes.
E. decreased body fat.

A............ B.......... C.......... D.......... E..........

467. A. T   B. T   C. T   D. T   E. T

At the start of glucocorticoid therapy, patients tend to have insomnia, increased appetite, weight gain or emotional lability. Hypertension, diabetes mellitus, acne vulgaris and peptic ulcer develop in those with risk factors. Prolonged and intense steroid therapy may result in Cushingoid habitus, osteonecrosis, suppression of the hypothalamic–pituitary–adrenal axis, increased susceptibility to infection, myopathy and impaired wound healing; these can be minimised by using conservative dosage regimens. Delayed and insidious complications are dependent on the cumulative dose and these include osteoporosis, atherosclerosis, growth retardation, skin atrophy, fatty liver and cataracts. Rare and unpredictable side-effects of steroid therapy include psychosis, pseudotumour cerebri, glaucoma, lipomatosis over the dura and pancreatitis.

468. A. T   B. T   C. T   D. T   E. F

Indications for pulse regimes for steroids include 1) Recrudescence of disease despite steroid therapy 2) Flare of disease activity in patients who have steroid side-effects. 3) The need to control disease until another treatment modality becomes effective. 4) The onset of rapidly progressive steroid-responsive syndrome.

469. A. F   B. F   C. F   D. T   E. F

Glomerular filtration rate diminishes with advancing age. However, many individuals are able to maintain near-normal glomerular filtration rate in late life. As the lean muscle mass (the source of creatinine) also declines with age, serum creatinine is not useful in predicting age-related decline in glomerular filtration rate. Formulas for rapid estimation of glomerular filtration rate have been validated in the elderly and should be used with drugs with a narrow therapeutic index, such as digoxin or aminoglycosides. Serum drug levels should be used to guide therapy in these patients. Hepatic blood flow may decrease with age, diminishing the efficiency of the liver to metabolise drugs. Oxidative processes (phase I metabolism) has been shown to decline with age in some studies, whereas hepatic conjugation (phase II metabolism) is unaltered with age. Unlike oxidised metabolites, which are often active, conjugated metabolites are usually inactive. Body fat increases with age, resulting in a lower volume of distribution for water-soluble drugs and a higher volume of distribution for fat-soluble drugs. As a result fat-soluble drugs may reach steady-state concentrations later than expected causing delayed toxicity, whereas the onset of water-soluble drugs may be sooner.

470. *In the elderly, presenting features of faecal impaction include*

    A. fever.
    B. altered mental status.
    C. agitation.
    D. urinary retention.
    E. paradoxical diarrhoea.

    A.......... B.......... C.......... D.......... E..........

471. *An 85-year-old patient with terminal cancer complained of constipation. Drugs that could have contributed to this include*

    A. tricyclic antidepressants.
    B. anticholinergics.
    C. calcium channel antagonists.
    D. opioid analgesics.
    E. magnesium-containing antacids.

    A.......... B.......... C.......... D.......... E..........

472. *The following statements about overactivity of the bladder detrusor are correct.*

    A. It is a rare cause of urinary incontinence in the elderly.
    B. The detrusor muscle contracts in response to inappropriately small volumes of urine.
    C. It is often preceded by a sense of urgency.
    D. Antispasmodic agents such as oxybutinin should be avoided.
    E. It is important to rule out 'overflow incontinence' due to urinary retention prior to embarking on treatment.

    A.......... B.......... C.......... D.......... E..........

473. *The following statements about stress incontinence are correct.*

    A. It is characteristically rare in elderly women.
    B. It occurs due to detrusor contraction.
    C. Exogenous oestrogens should be avoided in these patients.
    D. Chronic indwelling catheters are usually required in these patients.
    E. Chronic antibiotic therapy is essential in these patients.

    A.......... B.......... C.......... D.......... E..........

470. A. T   B. T   C. T   D. T   E. T

In the elderly faecal impaction may present with fever, altered mental status, agitation, urinary retention or paradoxical diarrhoea. Because of these presentations, faecal impaction can be mistaken for other problems, leading to inappropriate treatment. In extreme cases, mechanical bowel obstruction may occur, necessitating surgical intervention, but faecal impaction can usually be treated with suppositories, enemas or manual disimpaction. Prevention consists of strict attention to the patient's bowel habits, adequate hydration and adequate but not excessive dietary fibre, avoidance of constipating medications when possible, and judicious use of laxatives.

471. A. T   B. T   C. T   D. T   E. F

All the drugs except magnesium containing antacids cause constipation. Magnesium causes diarrhoea and is present in the milk of magnesia, a laxative.

472. A. F   B. F   C. T   D. F   E. T

Overactivity of the bladder detrusor is the most common cause of urinary incontinence in elderly men and women. In this condition (also called detrusor hyperreflexia or detrusor instability), the detrusor muscle contracts in response to inappropriate small volumes of urine, often preceded by a sense of urgency. Incontinence results if the patient is unable to get to the toilet on time or when other problems, such as uretheral incompetence or bladder inflammation, co-exist. The symptoms of detrusor overactivity – frequency and urge incontinence – may be ameliorated by 'bladder training', consisting of prolonging the interval between voidings using behavioural techniques. Patients who are physically disabled or cognitively impaired should be toileted frequently or on a schedule, and incontinence garments (adult diapers) may be used. Antispasmodic agents such as oxybutinin may be useful: this type of medication relaxes the bladder wall and promotes storage of urine, presumably by inhibiting cholinergically mediated detrusor contractions.

473. A. F   B. F   C. F   D. F   E. F

True stress incontinence typically occurs after a cough or sneeze or in severe cases merely upon arising from a sitting position. Pelvic and distal urethral tissue contain oestrogen and progesterone receptors, and the urethra may become patulous after menopause. Stress incontinence may respond to treatment with exogenous oestrogens, although controversy exists over the precise mode or site of action of these hormones. Chronic indwelling catheters should not be used in the management of incontinence. The prevalence of urinary tract infection is virtually 100% in chronically catheterised patients.

474. *Causes of acute urinary retention include*

    A. diuretic therapy.
    B. faecal impaction.
    C. disopyramide.
    D. tricyclic antidepressants.
    E. benign prostatic hyperplasia.

    A.......... B.......... C.......... D.......... E..........

475. *Causes of bone loss include*

    A. primary hyperparathyroidism.
    B. heparin therapy.
    C. cigarette smoking.
    D. excess alcohol intake.
    E. vitamin C deficiency.

    A.......... B.......... C.......... D.......... E..........

476. *The following statements about hip fractures are correct.*

    A. In the absence of a fall hip fracture is almost always due to torsion or increased loading on a severely osteopenic femoral neck.
    B. Initial radiographs sometimes fail to reveal a fracture.
    C. Even in medically stable patients surgery should be avoided in the first 24–48 h.
    D. Postoperative delirium is common.
    E. The incidence of hip fracture rises steadily after the age of 60.

    A.......... B.......... C.......... D.......... E..........

477. *Causes of hyponatraemia include*

    A. congestive cardiac failure
    B. enteral tube feeds.
    C. intravenous saline therapy.
    D. SIADH.
    E dehydration.

    A.......... B.......... C.......... D.......... E..........

474. A. T   B. T   C. T   D. T   E. T

Urinary retention in men is most often related to prostatic outlet obstruction due to benign prostatic hyperplasia. Acute urinary retention may occur in elderly men and less often in women as the result of faecal impaction, the bedridden state, immobility or anticholinergic drugs, such as tricyclic antidepressants, diisopyramide, first-generation antihistamines and drugs used to treat incontinence. Diuretics can also lead to urinary retention when they produce a volume of urine that overwhelms the compromised bladder. Urinary retention may develop following surgery; this at least partly due to prolonged effects of anaesthetic agents and opioid analgesics.

475. A. T   B. T   C. T   D. T   E. F

Preventable causes of bone loss such as primary hyperparathyroidism, vitamin D deficiency, phosphate depletion, use of corticosteroids, heparin, cigarette smoking, excessive alcohol intake and marginal calcium intake.

476. A. F   B. T   C. F   D. T   E. T

Some hip fractures probably occur before or in the absence of fall perhaps because of torsion or other increased loading upon a severely osteopenic femoral neck. Incidence of hip fracture rises steadily after the age of 60. Approximately 17% of men and over 30% of all women sustain a hip fracture by age 90. Initial radiographs sometimes fail to reveal a fracture. Surgery should be performed as soon as the patient is medically stabilised because morbidity and mortality rise exponentially if surgery is delayed beyond 24 to 48 hours.

477. A. T   B. T   C. F   D. T   E. F

Dehydration can lead to hypernatraemia, and in the elderly the thirst response to dehydration is diminished making it more likely for high sodium levels. Congestive heart failure, central neurologic impairments and SIADH cause hyponatraemia. Enteral tube feeding has frequently been associated with hyponatraemia. Although hypotonic feeds may be partly to blame, hyponatraemia in tube-fed patients may also be a marker for underlying central nervous system disease, which has been associated with SIADH. Serum sodium must be monitored in neurologically impaired tube-fed patients and attention paid to the amount of free water added or used to flush the feeding tube. When saline solutions are given to correct dehydration, salt deficits or fluid-electrolyte imbalance, they must be infused cautiously and with careful monitoring, as heart failure is more likely consequence in the elderly. The risk of congestive cardiac failure may be related to underlying cardiac disease, decreased left ventricular compliance or another age-related defect in sodium metabolism – the decreased ability of the kidney to excrete a sodium load.

478. *Pressure sores*

A. occur within the first 2 weeks of hospitalisation.
B. develop when extrinsic pressure on the skin falls below mean capillary pressure.
C. over the heel tend to heal readily.
D. can be prevented by sliding (instead of lifting) bed-ridden patients.
E. with ulcer craters are usually treated with topical antibiotics.

A.......... B.......... C.......... D.......... E..........

479. *Recognised features of dementia include*

A. significant impairment of short-term memory.
B. significant impairment of long-term memory.
C. significant impairment of judgement.
D. significant impairment of abstract thinking.
E. personality change.

A.......... B.......... C.......... D.......... E..........

480. *Recognised features of vitamin B_{12} deficiency include*

A. decreased vibration sense in the legs.
B. microcytic anaemia.
C. hypersegmentation of neutrophils.
D. anisocytosis.
E. basophilic stippling.

A.......... B.......... C.......... D.......... E..........

481. *The following statements about ethanol metabolism are correct.*

A. It is absorbed almost completely from the gastrointestinal tract.
B. Over 90% is metabolised in the kidneys, lung and skin.
C. Elimination follows zero-order kinetics.
D. Its oxidation by hepatic alcohol dehydrogenase is the rate-limiting step.
E. Alcoholic flush seen in Japanese individuals is due to increased activity of aldehyde dehydrogenase.

A.......... B.......... C.......... D.......... E..........

482. *Neurological manifestations of alcoholism include*

A. Wernicke–Korsakoff syndrome.
B. cerebral atrophy.
C. central pontine myelinolysis
D. Marchiafava–Bignami disease.
E. peripheral neuropathy.

A.......... B.......... C.......... D.......... E..........

478. A. T   B. F   C. F   D. F   E. F

Most pressure sores develop in elderly patients within the first 2 weeks of hospitalisation. They develop when the extrinsic pressure on the skin exceeds mean capillary pressure (about 32 mmHg) resulting in diminished blood flow and tissue oxygenation. In recumbent patients, pressures over the sacrum or greater trochanter can reach as high as 100–150 mmHg. Pressure sores over the heel are characteristically stubborn when accompanied by arterial insufficiency. In bed-ridden patients, pressure sores can be prevented by lifting (not sliding) while moving patients. Pressure sores with ulcer craters should not be treated with topical antibiotics as they promote antimicrobial resistance.

479. A. T   B. T   C. T   D. T   E. T

Dementia is characterised by significant impairment of short-term memory, long-term memory, judgement (as indicated by inability to make reasonable plans to deal with interpersonal, social and work-related problems) and abstract thinking (as indicated by difficulty in defining work and concepts previously known). Also associated is personality change, such as alteration or accentuation of premorbid traits.

480. A. T   B. F   C. T   D. T   E. T

In vitamin B12 deficiency the anaemia is macrocytic, there is decreased vibration sense in the legs, hypersegmentation of neutrophils, anisocytosis and basophilic stippling.

481. A. T   B. F   C. T   D. T   E. F

Ethanol is almost completely absorbed from the gastrointestinal tract; about 25% enters the bloodstream from the stomach and the remainder from the intestine. Factors that modify absorption include food, the type, amount and concentration of the alcohol beverage, the rate of drinking and alterations in gastrointestinal motility. Over 90% is metabolised in the liver with less than 2–10% excreted by the lungs, kidneys and skin. Elimination follows zero-order kinetics and is independent of concentration. The oxidation of ethanol to acetaldehyde by hepatic alcohol dehydrogenase is the rate-limiting step and accounts for over 90% of the ethanol metabolised *in vivo*. Acetaldehyde is converted to acetate by aldehyde dehydrogenase; mutations of this enzyme in 50% of Japanese and other people of Far Eastern extraction results in reduced enzyme activity *in vivo* and the affected individuals experience an alcoholic flush.

482. A. T   B. T   C. T   D. T   E. T

Recognised neurological manifestations of alcoholism include Wernicke's encephalopathy (opthalmoplegia, nystagmus confusion and neuropathy, Korsakoff's psychosis (recent memory loss and confabulation), cerebellar degeneration, Marchiafava-Bignami disease (symmetrical demyelination of corpus callosum), central pontine myelinolysis, ambylopia. epilepsy, myopathy and rhabdomyolysis.

483.   *In a 70-year-old alcoholic brought to the accident and emergency department in stupor and coma*

    A. endotracheal intubation should be avoided.
    B. intravenous dextrose should always be administered before thiamine.
    C. ketoacidosis is improved by administration of 5% dextrose in 0.5N (0.45%) saline.
    D. haemodialysis should be considered if the blood ethanol exceeds $600\,mg\,dl^{-1}$.
    E. lateralising neurological signs suggest urgent intracranial pathology and a CT scan should be performed immediately.

    A..........   B..........   C..........   D..........   E..........

484.   *Recognised features of alcohol withdrawal include*

    A. resistance to sedatives.
    B. tremulousness.
    C. auditory hallucinations.
    D. convulsions.
    E. hyperpyrexia.

    A..........   B..........   C..........   D..........   E..........

485.   *The following statements are correct.*

    A. Mode is the most common value.
    B. Gaussian distribution is where continuous variables are distributed in a bell-shaped fashion.
    C. When the variables are normally distributed the mean plus or minus two standard deviations contains 96% of the observed values.
    D. The standard error of the mean measures the precision of the mean itself.
    E. The standard error of the mean is always smaller than the standard deviation.

    A..........   B..........   C..........   D..........   E..........

483.   A. F   B. F   C. T   D. T   E. T

If a patient is stuporous and unable to walk, the airways should be evaluated immediately. Patients should have an endotracheal tube inserted if in coma, hypoventilating or accumulating secretions. The presence of lateralising neurological signs suggest urgent intracranial damage and a CT scan should be performed immediately. Routine CT scans in alcoholic intoxication are not indicated. Gastric lavage may be performed if stupor is due to recent massive ingestion, but only after endotracheal intubation. Haemodialysis should be considered if the blood ethanol exceeds $600\,mg\,dl^{-1}$. Alcoholic ketoacidosis is improved by administration of 5% dextrose in 0.5 N (0.45%) saline. Thiamine 100 mg should be given parenterally to prevent or treat Wernicke's encephalopathy. It should be administered before or with intravenous dextrose. Administration of dextrose without thiamine may precipitate Wernicke's encephalopathy, because the glucose load may exhaust the already-depleted thiamine stores in alcoholic patients.

484.   A. T   B. T   C. T   D. T   E. T

With abrupt cessation of drinking in alcoholics, the patients develop a hyperexcitable state and manifestations of this include tremulousness, disordered perception (particularly auditory hallucinations), convulsions and delirium tremens. Alcoholics undergoing withdrawal are very resistant to sedatives (cross-tolerance) and large doses are required to calm their agitation. Benzodiazepines are used to manage the symptoms. Over-sedation should be avoided as there is a danger of respiratory depression. Delirium tremens is an acute medical emergency requiring hospitalisation; it is complicated by a high mortality (15%), particularly when complicated by hyperpyrexia and dehydration.

485.   A. T   B. T   C. T   D. T   E. T

The mean is the average value and the standard error of the mean measures the precision of the mean itself; and it is not appropriate to use the standard error of the mean as a measure of dispersion. It is always smaller than the standard deviation. The mode is the most common value, whereas the median is the middle value or the 50th percentile. Normal or Gaussian distribution is where continuous variables are distributed in a bell-shaped fashion. When the variables are normally distributed the mean plus or minus two standard deviations contains 96% of the observed values.

486. *The following statements about the null hypothesis are correct.*

   A. The *P* value is the likelihood that an observed difference or an even more extreme difference is due to chance alone.
   B. A very low *P* value strongly suggests that observed data are inconsistent with the null hypothesis.
   C. A type 1 error is an error of rejecting a true null hypothesis.
   D. A type 2 error occurs when a large *P* value leads to the incorrect conclusion that a difference does not exist (i.e. incorrectly not rejecting a null hypothesis).
   E. A type 2 error occurs when the study lacks the statistical power to demonstrate a true association or difference.

   A.......... B.......... C.......... D.......... E..........

487. *The following statements are correct.*

   A. Serum cholesterol is elevated during pregnancy.
   B. Total serum protein concentration increases by one-fifth by mid pregnancy.
   C. Intrahepatic cholestasis of pregnancy usually appears in the first trimester.
   D. Acute fatty liver of pregnancy is associated with increased microvesicular fat.
   E. Thrombocytopenia in pregnancy is most often due to pre-eclampsia.

   A.......... B.......... C.......... D.......... E..........

488. *Anxiety is associated with the following physical diseases:*

   A. hyperthyroidism.
   B. phaeochromocytoma.
   C. hypoglycaemia.
   D. partial seizures.
   E. alcohol withdrawal.

   A.......... B.......... C.......... D.......... E..........

489. *Causes of delirium include*

   A. thiamine deficiency.
   B. hepatic failure.
   C. hypoglycaemia.
   D. anticonvulsant intoxication.
   E. alcohol withdrawal.

   A.......... B.......... C.......... D.......... E..........

486. A. T   B. T   C. T   D. T   E. T

The null hypothesis is one that has no effect and if the null hypothesis is true and a study is well designed then any observed difference between the two gaps will be due to random sampling. The P-value is the likelihood that an observed difference or an even more extreme difference is due to chance alone. A small P value prevents against chance leading use to reject a null hypothesis which is true. A very low P value strongly suggests that observed data are inconsistent with the null hypothesis. A type 1 error is an error of rejecting a true null hypothesis. A type 2 error occurs when a large P value leads to the incorrect conclusion that a difference does not exist (i.e. incorrectly not rejecting a null hypothesis). A type 2 error occurs when the study lacks the statistical power to demonstrate a true association or difference.

487. A. T   B. F   C. F   D. T   E. T

Thrombocytopenia in pregnancy is usually due to pre-eclampsia; other causes include sepsis and idiopathic thrombocytopenic purpura. In idiopathic thrombocytopenic purpura, anti-platelet antibodies may cross the placenta to cause thrombocytopenia in the fetus. Serum triglycerides and cholesterol are elevated during pregnancy. Intrahepatic cholestasis of pregnancy usually occurs in the third trimester and is manifested by pruritus and elevated serum alkaline phosphatase and bilirubin. The itching and cholestasis disappear following delivery but may recur in subsequent pregnancy; treatment is symptomatic. The acute fatty liver of pregnancy displays increased microvesicular fat and fibrin in the hepatic sinusoids, usually appears in late pregnancy and is associated with pre-eclampsia. It is associated with DIC and maternal mortality may occur. It is also usually ameliorated following delivery.

488. A. T   B. T   C. T   D. T   E. T

Anxiety is associated with all these conditions

489. A. T   B. T   C. T   D. T   E. T

Delirium is an impairment in consciousness accompanied by abnormalities and perception and can occur due to thiamine deficiency, hepatic failure, hypoglycemia, anticonvulsant intoxication and alcohol withdrawal.

490. *Drugs causing psychosis include*

   A. diazepam.
   B. glucocorticoids.
   C. digitalis.
   D. phenytoin.
   E. amantidine.

   A.......... B.......... C.......... D.......... E..........

491. *Unwanted effects of lithium therapy include*

   A. weight gain.
   B. non-toxic goitre.
   C. hypothyroidism.
   D. nephrogenic diabetes insipidus.
   E. ataxia.

   A.......... B.......... C.......... D.......... E..........

492. *Withdrawal syndrome with benzodiazepines includes*

   A. akathisia.
   B. insomnia.
   C. convulsions.
   D. anxiety.
   E. tardive dyskinesia.

   A.......... B.......... C.......... D.......... E..........

493. *Features of alcohol dependence syndrome include*

   A. a compulsive need to drink.
   B. a stereotyped pattern of drinking.
   C. drinking takes primacy over other activities.
   D. relief of symptoms by further drinking.
   E. tolerance to alcohol is altered.

   A.......... B.......... C.......... D.......... E..........

494. *Management of delirium tremens includes the following:*

   A. patients are treated on an outpatient basis.
   B. intravenous chlormethiazole is the drug of choice.
   C. thiamine should be avoided.
   D. any dehydration should be corrected.
   E. oral disulfiram.

   A.......... B.......... C.......... D.......... E..........

490. A. F   B. T   C. T   D. T   E. T

Glucocorticoids, digitalis, phenytoin and amantidine cause psychosis whereas diazepam is used to treat the psychosis.

491. A. T   B. T   C. T   D. T   E. T

Lithium therapy causes several side effects include weight gain, non-toxic goitre, hypothyroidism, nephrogenic diabetes insipidus and ataxia.

492. A. F   B. T   C. T   D. T   E. F

Insomnia, convulsions and anxiety are caused due to benzodiazepine withdrawal whereas as akathisia and tardive dyskinesia are side effects due to L-dopa.

493. A. T   B. T   C. T   D. T   E. T

Alcohol dependence syndrome is usually very much easier to identify than problem-related drinking. Features include subjective awareness of a compulsion to drink, a narrowing of the drinking repertoire, primacy of drinking over other activities, increased tolerance to alcohol, need for more alcohol to achieve the same results, withdrawal symptoms, bad nerves, shakiness and blackouts through to delirium tremens, relief from avoidance of withdrawal symptoms by further drinking, rapid reinstatement of syndrome on drinking after period of abstinence.

494. A. F   B. F   C. F   D. T   E. F

Management of delirium tremens includes hospitalization, oral chlormethiazole, any dehydration should be corrected, treatment of any systemic infection, parenteral vitamins include thiamine. Disulfiram (antabuse) should be avoided during delirium tremens.

495. *The following statements are correct.*

A. Glue sniffing can cause death.
B. Amphetamine causes physical rather than psychological dependence.
C. Cannabis causes a severe withdrawal syndrome.
D. LSD is hallucinogenic.
E. Physical dependence occurs with morphine.

A.......... B.......... C.......... D.......... E..........

496. *Conditions associated with narcotic addicts include*

A. infective endocarditis.
B. tuberculosis.
C. glomerulonephritis.
D. tetanus.
E. hepatitis B.

A.......... B.......... C.......... D.......... E..........

497. *Aetiological factors implicated in anorexia nervosa include*

A. disturbance of hypothalamic function.
B. a disturbance in body image.
C. dietary problems in early life.
D. overprotective relationships.
E. lack of conflict resolution.

A.......... B.......... C.......... D.......... E..........

498. *Features of bulimia nervosa include*

A. cardiac arrhythmias.
B. renal impairment.
C. tetany.
D. muscular paralysis.
E. eroded dental enamel.

A.......... B.......... C.......... D.......... E..........

499. *Medical conditions affecting sexual performance include*

A. angina pectoris.
B. alcoholic cirrhosis.
C. asthma.
D. renal failure.
E. neuropathy.

A.......... B.......... C.......... D.......... E..........

495. A. T   B. F   C. F   D. T   E. T

Glue sniffing is dangerous because inhaled vomit can lead to asphyxiation, risk of tissue damage including damage to bone marrow, brain, liver and kidneys. With amphetamines psychological rather than true physical dependence is the role. Cannabis has no definite withdrawal syndrome or tolerance. Lysergic acid diethylamide (LSD), cannabis and mescaline are hallucinogenic drugs that produce distortions and intensifications of sensory perceptions as well as frank hallucinations.

496. A. T   B. T   C. T   D. T   E. T

Infective endocarditis, tuberculosis, glomerulonephritis are common causes of death in narcotic addicts while tetanus, malaria and acute viral hepatitis B are also causally related to addiction.

497. A. T   B. T   C. T   D. T   E. T

Aetiological factors implicated in anorexia include genetic, disturbances of hypothalamic function, a disturbance of body image, dietary problems in early life, overprotective relationship, rigidity and lack of conflict resolution.

498. A. T   B. T   C. T   D. T   E. T

Features of bulimia nervosa include self-induced vomiting, laxative abuse, misuse of diuretics, thyroid extracts or anorectics, consequences of low potassium (cardiac arrhythmias, renal impairment, muscular paralysis), hypokalemic paralysis (tetany), consequences of vomiting (swollen salivary glands, eroded enamel), fluctuations in body weight, irregular menstruation and neurotic personality traits.

499. A. T   B. T   C. T   D. T   E. T

Medical conditions affecting sexual performance include 1) Endocrine: Diabetes mellitus, hyperthyroidism, hypothyroidism 2) Cardiovascular: Angina pectoris, previous myocardial infarction, disorders of peripheral circulation 3) Hepatic: Alcohol related cirrhosis 4) Renal Failure 5) Neurological: Neuropathy, spinal cord lesions 5) Arthritis 6) Respiratory: Asthma, Chronic bronchitis and emphysema.

500. *Drugs adversely affecting sexual arousal include*

   A. cimetidine.
   B. alcohol.
   C. methyldopa.
   D. clonidine.
   E. benzodiazepines.

   A...........   B..........   C..........   D..........   E..........

500.   A. T   B. T   C. T   D. T   E. T

Drugs adversely affecting sexual arousal in males include alcohol, benzodiazepines, neuroleptics, cimetidine, narcotic analgesics, methyldopa, clonidine, spironolactone and antihistamines. Drugs adversely affecting sexual arousal in females include alcohol, CNS depressants, oral combined contraceptives, methyldopa and clonidine.